To my husband, John:

Over the past fifteen years you have given me so much. Thank you for showing me how to be a better person by example. Your consistent love, support and encouragement has propelled my purpose in Christ.

There were times when your words and actions were so unselfish until I was left in awe. Sharing my life with you has helped develop my character in ways that I would not have experienced without your temperance. Thank you for being my friend, lover and husband.

Yours forever,
Ruby

DIABETES WILL STOP WITH ME

"USING THE KINGDOM PRESCRIPTION"

RUBY MCMILLIAN

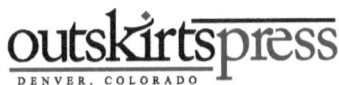

outskirtspress

DENVER, COLORADO

Acknowledgements

Reverend Ruby McMillian

I met this amazing woman of God in 1989, I was 27 years old with a 3-month-old baby boy. This was a very trying time in my life because I was homeless and five months clean from a drug addition to crack cocaine. But for the grace of God! She came into my life, and how amazing was that within itself...

I was in a rehabilitation program for mothers with children. This was a short term program so after three months, it was time for me to move on. I didn't have anywhere to go because everybody in the life I left behind was either on drugs, in jail from drugs, or had already passed away from using or selling drugs. Yes, including my parents.

There was a lady who had recently started a faith-based transitional housing program. At that time, faith-based meant no funding from the government. Before this point in my life, I hadn't known any "Real" Christian people. The kind of religion I knew was the kind where people get dressed up on Easter morning go to church and sin the rest of the year until Easter comes round again.

This lady came to pick me up and when she came, it was as if she had known me all my life. She was beautiful, confident and she stood very tall. I was enamored with her poise and grace. She didn't ask me a lot of questions, she wasn't judging me. For the first time in my life, I felt like everybody else—just me.

She took me to this beautiful home in the city of Hercules, California. We walked in the door and she said to me "Welcome home." I tried to hold back the tears that were welling up in my eyes. Consider a person with no family support, homeless with a little baby and two other children that were sent to another state for a time to be with their relatives because I could not properly care for them. I was a mess!

This beautiful woman taught me how to cook, clean, and be productive. Most importantly, she taught me that I was somebody and that God loved me. She was actually the first person who ever really believed in me and taught me that I could do ALL things through Christ who strengthens me.

Like I said before, she is very beautiful, however, when I first met her, she was also a bit overweight. I guess that came along with all that delicious southern comfort food she used to cook. After leaving her program, some time went by before we re-connected. She came over to my home in Fremont, California and I hardly recognized her. She was slim and so healthy looking. I asked her what happened and she told me that she was diagnosed a diabetic and she had to make some changes in her life.

She told me that she had learned how to read her lab blood work and how to use this very unique breathing technique combined with some stretching exercises that looked strange and funny. After seeking God in prayer for guidance, he had given her something amazing called the "Kingdom Prescription Lifestyle." A woman in her 50s, she was too gorgeous inside and out. I asked her to show me this technique.

WOW! What a rush to the brain. So deep breathing can oxygenate your blood to make your body burn fat, clear up and improve your mind and give you a body shaped like that? I thought before that you were poised but this you really shows an even more confident quality of life. O.K. I want it too.

She is my true American Hero. I really could go on and on about this amazing, anointed, gift from God but for the purposes of this writing, I will stop for now.

--Sharon Tracee Cowart

Contents

Preface

Dear Family and New Readers:

I have written this book to teach each of you how to prayerfully and practically move through making the changes necessary to rid your body of Type 2 Diabetes. It has been at epidemic status for decades in our churches and especially in the African American families.

God answered my cry when I sought him for answers about my body being afflicted with Type 2 Diabetes. By the time you have completely read this book, you too will be radically changed.

For five years this "Kingdom Prescription" has kept my A1 C count within normal limits. My doctor asked if she could share my methods with other patients because my results have been proven year after year.

It is God's desire for all men and women to be in good health and prosper as their souls prosper. You will prosper as you read how these revelations can change your life forever. So get a cup of your favorite drink, take your comfy position as you join me on this personal journey to learn how to put Type-2 Diabetes to death in your body.

Blessings and Health,
Ruby Moorer-McMillian

Introduction

It has taken me almost four decades to write these truths. I did not write this book to overwhelm you, but rather to compel you to change one thing at a time.

By taking this approach you will feel and acknowledge the effect it has on your body. By using these practical but surprisingly simple methods you are going to change your mind about never becoming healthy again without dieting forever. Your vision of how you see yourself will never be the same either. As you commit to giving yourself a 15-minute "Breath of Life Treatment" you will notice a surge of warmth coming over your body.

You will have more energy to get you started daily. But more importantly, you will have more energy at the end of the day too. Diseases will have to rest and cease to exist after their encounter with the "Breath of Life" treatments.

Cleansing your body's bloodstream daily with the "Breath of Life" treatments will guarantee you a more vibrant inner self. Add the gifts of movement that God has given you to enjoy; this will accelerate the strengthening and toning of your body. Go ahead and get ready to experience the best you now!

Take a full five minutes and close your eyes and go into the theater of your mind and see yourself as the man or woman you want to become. Know this truth, "as a person thinks in their heart so is he or she."

As you read this powerful "Kingdom Prescription" your mind will be infused with revelations of how God has already given us what we need to break the curse of premature death. Now is your time to reclaim your youth. Reclaim your vitality. Claim your "Divine Health." Get ready to experience the lifestyle that you thought you had missed. But by the grace of God you have gotten this little book with the answers that will bring healing to your body within weeks.

Get ready for a new you without a "Diet Lifestyle." Because diets don't work! Using the Kingdom Prescription you will have a healthier body from the inside out once and for all. Yes, this method will give you the keys to a lifetime of great health.

When you put these powerful ingredients together:: reading the Word of God, praying the Word of God over your body daily, learning your blood work numbers,, use the deep breathing methods, select and eat super foods, taking the best supplements and using the gifts of movement daily,it will make you whole again. Soon you too will share your testimony of how the Kingdom Prescription saved your life from the dreaded disease of diabetes.

CHAPTER 1

Diabetes and Kidney Disease

Diabetes is a metabolic disease in which a person has a high blood sugar either because the pancreas doesn't produce insulin or cells do not respond to insulin that is produced. Diabetes is the leading cause of kidney failure, accounting for 44% of new cases each year and 35% of all cases in the U.S. Uncontrolled or poorly controlled high blood pressure is the 2nd leading cause of chronic kidney disease, accounting for 23% of cases. Overuse of common drugs such as Tylenol, Ibuprofen, and Aspirin can cause chronic kidney disease. The state of Alabama ranks 5th in the nation for kidney disease. Nearly 8000 Alabamians are receiving dialysis. One in every eight Americans have been diagnosed with chronic kidney disease. Some symptoms of diabetes include increased hunger, thirst, and frequent urination.

African Americans have the highest health risk of all cultural groups. African Americans have more diseases, disabilities, and early death as well. The lack of health care, the lack of trust in the medical system, cultural differences, problem accessing care, and the lack of knowledge about the importance of routine checkups and screenings contributes to poor health conditions.

Uncontrolled diabetes damages the kidneys. The kidneys are a bean-shaped organ located near the middle of the back. The kidneys remove toxins and waste from the bloodstream. Every day, the functioning kidney processes 200 quarts of blood to sift out two quarts of waste products and extra water which becomes urine. The kidneys also produce three hormones. One is renin, which helps regulate blood pressure. Another hormone is erythropoietin, which is used for the production of red blood cells.

Calcitriol is a third hormone excreted by the kidneys which helps maintain calcium for bones and chemical balance.

If a diabetic continues to have high blood glucose, the glucose stays in the bloodstream and acts as a poison which causes damage to the nephrons, which are the functioning unit of the kidneys. Controlling and managing your diabetes can prevent diabetic kidney disease.

There are different stages of kidney failure. Stage 1 is the mildly diminished function with few symptoms. In stages 2 and 3 the symptoms are getting progressively worse, and the person is treated by a nephrologist to slow down the diminished function of the kidney with treatment of the renal failure. Stages 4 and 5 are the severe stage. This patient is prepared to receive active treatment to survive. Stage 5 is the last stage of kidney failure. The patient must receive dialysis to prolong life.

Some signs and symptoms of renal failure include: vomiting,

diarrhea, nausea, weight loss, blood in the urine, shortness of breath and edema. Dialysis is the process of removing waste and excess water from the blood and is used for the artificial replacement of the lost kidney. Most patients have to dialyze three times a week an average three to five hours a day. These individuals must have an access in place to receive dialysis. There are different types of access used to receive dialysis such as fistulas, grafts, and vascular catheters.

Patients begin to feel better within the first week of dialysis. Some patients may exhibit some cramping or nausea and vomiting during treatment. These symptoms can be resolved by addressing the cause and effect, and educating the patient on fluid gains. The best prevention for a diabetic is to control their blood glucose, maintain a healthy diet, and have routine checkups by the Endocrinologist. The facts can help prevent kidney disease.

CHAPTER 2

The Kingdom Prescription

THE BLOOD

In ninety days you can change the amount of sugar that is being absorbed into your bloodstream. That's right, you can and will take control of the amount of sugar by eating less of these: desserts, breakfast cereal, candy bars and ice cream, starchy foods, and fried foods that will register overload in your blood. Here is what you have to do:

First, ask your doctor to order your blood work for a complete metabolic panel. These tests will give you a complete and accurate account of your metabolic blood numbers. Your blood is your body's' lifeline to divine health. Fondly, I like to call it my "Diagnostic Report." This test will give you an accurate account of your blood sugars and cholesterol numbers. One specific aspect of the panel is called your hemoglobin (A1C). This test gives the doctor your total blood sugar count over the past three months (90 days).

Once your test results are in sit down with your doctor and go over the test. Ask your physician to point out for you all the areas that are out of "normal range." Another example is your HGB A1C number. If your blood work test results are 6.5 and above those numbers are too high. The normal ranges are 4.1-6.4.

Plan of Action:

- Go to your doctor and get the blood work done.

- After you have gotten the results from your doctor go to the back of this book and write out your goal for the next thirty days.

- Follow the doctor's orders. Test your blood sugars as instructed.

- Give your body a 24-hour cleansing. Use a good colon cleanser. (Ask your doctor to recommend one). You can buy an over-the-counter cleanser. .

- Use only "clear liquids" for 24 hours. (Do one x every month)

- Give your body the gift of cleansing and resting your major organs.

- Drink as much of these as you desire:

- Low-sodium chicken broth, white grape juice, apple juice (no pulp) orange juice (no pulp) green tea, lots of gelatins (no red or purple gelatins). I suggest sugar-free only.

- No dairy /Non-dairy products. Coffee black with small amounts of honey or Agave as sweeteners. Drink plenty of water.

- Read the Word of God during this cleansing. Pray for the change in your appetite and a new reverence for your body (temple).

  Put on "soaking music." Receive fresh insights and thoughts from reading and praying the Word of God.

- Day Two: NEW BEGINNINGS-"Kingdom Lifestyle Eating"

- Prepare stir-fry meals. (Turn to the food preparation section).

- Make yourself huge green leaf salads with red, yellow or green bell peppers, tomatoes, red onions, cucumbers, shredded mix-cheeses, boiled egg, broccoli florets and mushrooms. Top it with or put on the side grilled, baked or blackened chicken, lamb chops, fish or turkey burgers.

- Purchase some fresh fruits that are in season.

- Purchase yourself some unsalted nuts. These are great for snacks with a big apple.

- Hydrate your body with plenty of water and melons.

- Remember what you put into your body (temple) will yield the results in your blood sugar diagnostic test in the next 90 days.

Kingdom Lifestyle "Eating every Word that proceeds out of the mouth of God"

1 Cor. 6: 12 (AMP) says this, *"Everything is permissible (allowable and lawful) for me; but not all things are helpful (good for me to do, expedient and profitable* *when considered with other things). Everything is lawful for me, but I will not become a slave of anything or be brought under its power.*

1 Cor. 6: 13a (AMP) says, *"Food (is intended) for the stomach and the stomach for the food."*

1 Cor. 6: 19-20 (AMP)

Do you not know that your body is the temple (the very sanctuary) of the Holy Spirit who lives within you, whom you have received (as a gift) from God? You are not your own.

You were bought with a price (purchased with a preciousness and paid for, made His own). So then, honor God and bring glory to Him in your body.

CHAPTER 3

Planning Strategies

1. Make it simple to follow. (Prepare three different dishes/ mix them up over five days).

2. Choose your meals for the next five days.

3. First, select your five breakfast meals.

4. Second, select the lunch meals.

5. Third, select your dinners for the next five days. (Prepare three meats. Mix them up as desired over the next five days).

6. Place it in the kitchen so you can see it.

7. Weekends are your options to choose what fits you without indulging in sugary desserts, white starchy foods and almost anything made with white flour.

8. Daily, prepare your selections and add beauty to the way you arrange the food on the dish. After all, you are royalty!

DESIGN YOUR BODY

1. Here you are designing your body by what you give it. Cooking and preparing for success is exciting.

2. You have a goal to see your numbers change.

3. Find or form a support person or group. This will help you stay focused and committed to make the change.

4. You are going to feel so good.

Now that you have the "kingdom meal planning" in control, let's move to the second aspect of your makeover.

[Insightful Nugget] The pirit of gluttony defined: This is the inability to have discipline over your stomach. Being unable to resist foods in excess of what is sufficient and proper for your body. Do not go to "all you can eat" establishments for the first 90 days.

THE BREATHS OF LIFE: (Isotonic Breathing)

This technique is simple, effective and it does look strange.

Defined: Pull hard breaths through your nostrils. Then open your mouth and push the breath out through your mouth. Then close your mouth again and hold your breath for the count of 5, 8 to 12, then the release. (you will hear a pop-like sound.)

Here is a video that will help you: www.bodyflex.com

GET UP 30 MINUTES EARLIER.

Take 10-15 deep isotonic breaths every morning. (On an empty stomach). Energy!

Take 10-15 deep isotonic breaths in the afternoon. (On an empty stomach) Energy!

Isometric Stretch during your Isotonic breathing. This allows the oxygenated blood to flow very rapidly through your arteries/ circulatory system and it washes the area of muscles that are stretched.

(Insightful Nugget) You may want to start this on a weekend because you need time to try it. You will laugh at it too. You will become more comfortable with practice. Also you will be able to do 10 or 15 breaths easily. You are going to feel warm as you oxygenate your blood. This breath of life technique is going to start changing you from the inside out. Deep breathing will give your blood an instant boost that does not cost you anything. But it will give your vital organs everything in exchange for a breath.

(Key) Oxygen is one of the most vital aspects of a healthy life. Use it as a fat-burning fuel, use it to heal, cleanse and revitalize your being!

Take Your Daily Supplements:

1. Chromium Picolinate 200 mgs. Start with (2) 200 mgs. tablets with meals two times per day. (In your journal keep a record of your intake of Chromium Picolinate for a week.) Record how you feel. Adjust if needed.

2. Magnesium 500 Mgs. One time per day with meal.

3. Calcium- with Vitamin D 1200 mgs. One time per day with meal.

4. Omega-3 Fish Oil 360 mgs. capsules. Take one per day with meal. (may use Cod-Liver Oil Caps. 1000 mgs.)

5. Ginseng 500 mgs. tablets or capsules. Take one tablet/capsule two times per day with meals. (A.M. and afternoon, preferably 2-4 p.m.)

6. Aloe Vera liquid is taken in your favorite juice. Add 6 ozs. Of Aloe Vera juice to four ozs. of your favorite juice.

7. Multi-Vitamin (Select the one that is right for your age).

   [Note: If you need iron-use the chelated or slow iron to retard constipation].

8. Apple cider vinegar and honey cocktail: Mix one teaspoon of apple cider vinegar in four oz.to six ozs. of water at room temperature with ½ teaspoon of pure honey or agave nectar. Stir well and drink five to fifteen minutes before your meal.

   (NOTE) This cocktail is designed to take before you eat a holiday meal, a meal high in fatty food or a meal that includes a larger than usual sugar intake on "Special Occasions." If you are sensitive to acid in the stomach you might want to just use the Chromium Picolinate.

9. Cinnamon 200 mgs./500 mgs. Take one capsule one time per day with dinner meal. (Insightful Nugget) Do not take cinnamon and bittet melon capsules together.

PLEASE try one over a period of 30 days to determine which one works best for you. 10. Bitter Melon 450 mgs. capsules. Take one capsule in the a.m. and one in p.m.The Gifts Of Movement

What Is Your Style?

We all have a few moves we love to make. Here is your opportunity to do them until you get enough.

- Choose your style of walking for 30 minutes per day. (Ex. Speed Walking-Use music it helps.)

- Choose to dance for one hour per day. Do it three to four times per week. (Get your Praise On)

- Choose an activity that you love. Mix it up so you will always look forward to an enjoyable committed "Regular Body Movement."

- Remember that a body in motion is forever toned, strong, resistant to most common illnesses and your mindset will become receptive to illuminating thoughts.

- Swimming is one of the most full-bodied cardio workouts ever.

- Biking/Cycling is how you want to roll.

- Running is an excellent way to get your stamina up.

- Early morning is a good time when it is cool and quiet after prayer.

—∞—

(Insightful Nugget) We were designed and made by God to praise Him in the dance.

CALLANETICS

(Callanetics) small intense body movements that work at tightening and strengthening all of your muscles. It will give you a very tight body. www.callanetics.com

You can get the body you want with little impact on your joints. I combine the two. Breathe before I do the move- Count to 12 –exhale- continue to finish my count. AMAZING!

FOOD PREPARATIONS

"Kingdom Lifestyle"

Stir-fry cooking: Use large skillet or wok. Place on burner and get hot; add three to five tablespoons of Sesame Seed Oil or Olive Oil.

Place your clean, washed vegetables in a cut up style that you enjoy . Use natural seasonings, Mrs. Dash, sea salt and fresh ground black or white pepper.

Meats for stir-fry: wash your raw chicken (skinless) and cut into nice slices. Raw turkey, do the same. Raw beef cut very thin; it will enable it to cook faster with more flavor.

Here are a few websites that will be helpful :

- www.mifoods.cm
- www.allrecipes,com/seasme-shrimp-stirfry
- www.foodnetwork.com
- www.youtube.com

Four Major Areas of Observation for Type - 2 Diabetes Prevention:

(DISCLAIMER: PLEASE CONSULT YOUR DOCTOR BEFORE MAKING MAJOR CHANGES TO YOUR DIET AND MEDICATIONS.)

A. YOUR BLOOD WORK NUMBERS

B. YOUR FOOD INTAKE CHOICES/SUPPLEMENTS

C. YOUR REGULAR CHOICE OF MOVEMENT/EXERCISE/ BREATHING/STRETCHING

D. READING AND CONFESSING THE WORD OF GOD OVER YOUR BODY.

1. BLOOD WORK:

KNOW YOUR OWN NUMBERS. KNOW WHAT YOUR BODY NEEDS TO FUNCTION AT ITS OPTIMUM CAPACITY.

DO IT FOR 90 DAYS. ASK YOUR DOCTOR TO EXPLAIN TO YOU WHAT IS OUT OF NORMAL LIMITS IN YOUR BLOODSTREAM.

2. FOOD CHOICES:

START YOUR DAY OFF WITH A GREAT BREAKFAST.TAKE PROPER SUPPLEMENTS WITH YOUR MEALS. EAT THREE BALANCED MEALS A DAY WITH TWO ENERGY SNACKS INSTEAD OF THREE WRONG ONES. GET PROPER REST (SEVEN TO EIGHT HOURS OF SLEEP PER DAY).

EAT GREEN AND YELLOW VEGGIES. EAT FRUIT- IF IT CAN BE TOLERATED.

LET GO OF THE DEEP FRIED MEATS. TRY OVEN FRIED INSTEAD. STOP USING FOODS HIGH IN STARCHES ON A REGULAR BASIS. SAVE THEM FOR SPECIAL OCCASIONS. USE LOTS OF FRESH VEGETABLES. STIR -FRY IN OLIVE OIL. USE LOTS OF NATURAL FRUITS AND VEGETABLES TO SATISFY THAT SWEET TOOTH. USE AGAVE NECTAR OR HONEY FOR YOUR SWEETENERS

TRY DOUBLE BAKED SWEET POTATOES/CARROT CASSEROLE.

USE LOTS OF HERBAL SEASONING. DRINK LOTS OF WATER DAILY. LARGE QUANTITIES OF WHITE SUGAR AND STARCHY FOODS ARE DIRECT KILLERS OF YOUR PANCREAS AND KIDNEYS.

SUPPLEMENTS: WHY USE THEM? OUR BODIES OFTEN DON'T PRODUCE

ENOUGH. A NUMBER OF OUR SUPPLEMENTS ARE WATER SOLUBLE. THEREFORE THEY NEED TO BE REPLACED DAILY.

HERE ARE THE SUPPLEMENTS THAT CAN MAKE A DIFFERENCE IMMEDIATELY IN YOUR HEALTH. THESE ARE THE SUPPLEMENTS THAT I HAVE PERSONALLY USED TO HELP MY BODY RID ITSELF OF THOSE SUDDEN FEELINGS OF BEING SICK, SWEATY AND SHAKY DUE TO MY BLOOD SUGAR DROPPING. IT IS ALSO CALLED HYPOGLYCEMIA.

1. CHROMIUM: A TRACE MINERAL THAT MIMICS INSULIN BY HELPING THE BODY PRODUCE MORE.

2. MAGNESIUM: A MINERAL THAT HELPS PROMOTE A HEALTHY PANCREAS. IT ALSO HELPS STOP BAD LEG CRAMPS.

3. CALCIUM-WITH VITAMIN D: GREAT FOR HELPING YOU HAVE STRONG BONES AND TEETH.

4. COD-LIVER OIL: IT IS THE BEST "FAT BUSTER" OF THOSE FATTY TRIGLYCERIDES

   IN THE BLOOD CELLS, IT ALSO HELPS LOWER YOUR

   BLOOD PRESSURE. IN ADDITION, IT IS GOOD FOR THE BRAIN, EYES AND YOU WILL MAINTAIN A BETTER MOOD.

5. MULTI-VITAMIN: THEY HELP YOU HAVE BETTER BLOOD SUGAR LEVELS.

   (ESPECIALLY GOOD FOR DIABETICS THAT ARE OVERWEIGHT)6. GINSENG: AN ANCIENT ORIENTAL ENDURANCE MINERAL. IT HELPS YOU THINK WITH MORE CLARITY. BALANCED ENERGY AND STAMINA.

7. ALOE VERA: ONE OF GOD'S MULTI-PURPOSE PLANTS. IT HELPS YOUR BODY'S

   IMMUNE SYSTEM AND HELP KEEPS YOUR BLOOD SUGARS LEVEL. IT AIDS YOUR BODY IN ATTACKING UNHEALTHY BACTERIA. IT CAN BE USED TO HEAL YOUR SORES, CLEARS UP ITCHY SCALP AND ITCHY SKIN.

8. CINNAMON: HAS BEEN RECOGNIZED TO HELP KEEP YOUR BLOOD SUGAR BALANCED NATURALLY BY USING A TEASPOON IN YOUR FOOD DAILY.

9. APPLE CIDER VINEGAR AND HONEY COCKTAIL: TWO-FER ONE OF THE BEST COMBINATIONS TO COMBAT FAT, STRESS, AND BLOOD SUGAR SPIKES AFTER EATING AND CLEARING UP YOUR SKIN IN THE PROCESS. (MIX ONE TEASPOON OF CIDER VINEGAR IN 4 0ZS. OF ROOM

   TEMPERATURE WATER WITH ONE ½ TEASPOON OF PURE HONEY. STIR WELL AND DRINK TEN TO FIIFTEEN MINUTES BEFORE A MEAL.)

3. REGULAR BODY MOVEMENT:

THERE MUST BE A REGULAR COMMITTED FORM OF GIVING YOUR BODY 45 MINUTES PER DAY. A MINIMUM OF FOUR TIMES PER WEEK AT 45 MINUTES. IT WIll CHANGE YOUR WAISTLINE, YOUR HEART RATE AND GIVE YOU HIGHER LEVELS OF ENERGY. CHOOSE YOUR MOVEMENTS. DO YOU LIKE TO DEEP BREATHING/BODY FLEX AND CALLANETICS=STRETCHING BIKING, SPEED WALKING, SWIMMING, DANCING, FLOOR EXERCISES OR TREADMILLS. IMMEDATE BENEFITS ARE NO MORE CONSTIPATION!

4. THE WORD OF GOD: USE THE WORD OF GOD AS YOUR DAILY CONFESSION REGARDING YOUR HEALTH.

A. 3 JOHN 2, SAYS THIS TO THE BELIEVER: "BELOVED, I WISH ABOVE ALL THINGS THAT THOU MAY PROSPER AND BE IN HEALTH, EVEN AS THY SOUL PROSPERS."

B. 1COR. 6:19-20 IS FOR THE BELIEVER. "KNOW YE NOT THAT YOUR BODY IS THE TEMPLE OF THE HOLY GHOST WHICH IS IN YOU, WHICH YOU HAVE OF GOD, AND YE ARE NOT YOUR OWN? V. 20 SAYS, FOR YOU WERE BOUGHT WITH A PRICE; THEREFORE GLORIFY GOD IN YOUR BODY AND IN YOUR SPIRIT, WHICH ARE GOD'S."

C. USE THE WORD OF GOD WITH EVERY CHANGE YOU MAKE IN YOUR LIFE TO KEEP YOU FOCUSED AND TO EXPERIENCE VICTORY.

D. PLAY SOME SOAKING MUSIC WHILE IN HIS PRESENCE, SET THE ATMOSPHERE.

E. I HAVE PROVIDED THIRTY SCRIPTURE DECLARATIONS TO HELP YOU GET STARTED.

THIS IS THE BEGINNING OF A BRAND NEW LIFE-STYLE!

YOUR BODY IS GOD'S IMAGE OF HIS DIVINE DESIGN. ALWAYS TREAT IT WITH THE RESPECT, GRACE AND THE CARE IT DESERVES. DON'T POUR SUGAR IN THE TANK. PUT IN PURE LIQUID GOLD INSTEAD. GIVE YOUR BODY PURE WATER, GREEN TEA, VITAMIN AND MINERALS, LEAN MEATS, GARDEN RAINBOW OF VEGGIES AND BLEND SWEET FRUITS WITH AGAVE OR HONEY TO MAKE A MOUTH-WATERING DESSERT.

THE KINGDOM PRESCRIPTION IS A LIFESTYLE MADE FOR GOD'S PEOPLE. HE HAS PRESCRIBED US A LIFE THAT IS HEALTHY AND FULL OF PASSION AND PURPOSE. THIS IS NOT A DIET! START WHERE YOU ARE WITH WANTING TO MAKE CHANGES. ONE THING IS FOR SURE, YOU WILL FEEL AMAZING!

A WORD FOR THE MEN: DECIDE NOW TO TAKE YOUR LOVE LIFE BACK! NOTE: APPROXIMATELY 90% OF MEN TAKING MEDICATION FOR HIGH BLOOD PRESSURE AND

DIABETES ARE EXPERIENCING ERECTILE DYSFUNCTION. BY USING THE KINGDOM PRESCRIPTION YOU WILL RESTORE THE BLOOD FLOW NATURALLY.

GET YOUR GROOVE BACK, MAKE YOUR WIFE A HAPPY WOMAN. DON'T LET THE PRESCRIPTION MEDICATION ROB YOU OF YOUR MARRIAGE BED THRILLS. IN A LITTLE AS 90 DAYS, YOU WILL BE WELL ABLE. YOU WILL HAVE MORE ENERGY, STRENGTH, AND DESIRE TO HONOR YOUR BODY AS GOD'S TEMPLE. FATIGUE WILL BE GONE FOREVER. YOU CAN HAVE IT ALL FOR A LONG, PASSIONATE AND SEXUALLY ENJOYABLE LIFESTYLE AGAIN. EXPERIENCE MORE YOUTHFULNESS AND LESS FATIGUE.

IT IS MY DIRECTIVE TO HELP THOSE WHO DESIRE TO BE HEALTHIER, HAPPIER AND LOOK

FORWARD TO ACCOMPLISHING THEIR MISSION IN "DIVINE HEALTH".

CONFIDENTIAL LABORATORY REPORT **LabCorp**
Laboratory Corporation of America

VERIFICATION

CHART:	Fasting:	DATE: 10/13/2004
PATIENT NAME:	MCMILLIAN, RUBY	SSN:
DOB:	08-11-	AGE:	SEX: F

FILLER ORD NO:	28658901640 LAB	SPECIMEN DATE:	10/12/2004
PHYSICIAN:	DOUGLAS, A	PHY ID:	DOUGLAS

TESTS	RESULT	FLAG	UNITS	REF. INTERVAL	LAB
HEMOGLOBIN A1C (FINAL)					
A1c	6.5 H		%	4.5-5.7	OM
Please note:	SPRCS				OM

Current guidelines recommend a treatment goal of <7% for diabetic patients. A1c may be overestimated in diabetic patients exhibiting poor control and who are also heterozygous or homozygous for HgbS or HgbC. Total glycohemoglobin is a better indicator of diabetic control in patients with these hemoglobin variants.

GLUCOSE, SERUM (FINAL)					
Glucose, Serum		113 H	mg/dL	65-99	OM

OM	Providence Med Grp DBA Mobile	PHONE	CONTACT	DIRECTOR
	6701 Airport Blvd Ste A101	(251) 633-8880		G Divittori MD
	Mobile, AL 366080000			

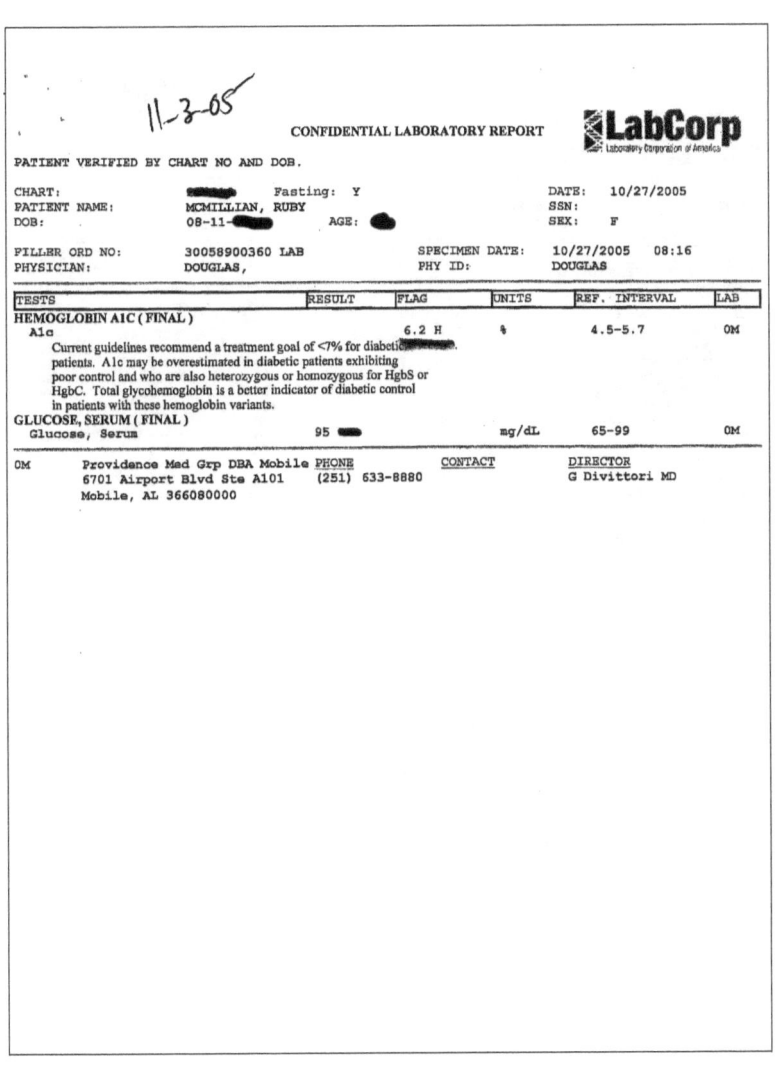

11-3-05

CONFIDENTIAL LABORATORY REPORT

LabCorp
Laboratory Corporation of America

PATIENT VERIFIED BY CHART NO AND DOB.

CHART:	⬛ Fasting: Y	DATE:	10/27/2005
PATIENT NAME:	MCMILLIAN, RUBY	SSN:	
DOB:	08-11-⬛ AGE: ⬛	SEX:	F

FILLER ORD NO:	30058900360 LAB	SPECIMEN DATE:	10/27/2005 08:16
PHYSICIAN:	DOUGLAS,	PHY ID:	DOUGLAS

TESTS	RESULT	FLAG	UNITS	REF. INTERVAL	LAB
HEMOGLOBIN A1C (FINAL)					
A1c	6.2 H	%	4.5-5.7	OM

Current guidelines recommend a treatment goal of <7% for diabetic ⬛ patients. A1c may be overestimated in diabetic patients exhibiting poor control and who are also heterozygous or homozygous for HgbS or HgbC. Total glycohemoglobin is a better indicator of diabetic control in patients with these hemoglobin variants.

TESTS	RESULT	FLAG	UNITS	REF. INTERVAL	LAB
GLUCOSE, SERUM (FINAL)					
Glucose, Serum	95 ⬛		mg/dL	65-99	OM

OM	Providence Med Grp DBA Mobile PHONE	CONTACT	DIRECTOR
	6701 Airport Blvd Ste A101 (251) 633-8880		G Divittori MD
	Mobile, AL 366080000		

CONFIDENTIAL LABORATORY REPORT

≋LabCorp
Laboratory Corporation of America

PATIENT VERIFIED BY CHART NO AND DOB.

CHART:	▮▮▮▮, Fasting: Y	DATE:	11/09/2005
PATIENT NAME:	MCMILLIAN, RUBY	SSN:	
DOB:	08-11-▮▮▮ AGE: ▮▮	SEX:	F

FILLER ORD NO:	31358900250 LAB	SPECIMEN DATE:	11/09/2005	08:04
PHYSICIAN:	DOUGLAS,	PHY ID:	DOUGLAS	

TESTS	RESULT	FLAG	UNITS	REF. INTERVAL	LAB
COMP. METABOLIC PANEL (14) (FINAL)					
Glucose, Serum	92		mg/dL	65-99	OM
BUN	12		mg/dL	5-26	OM
Creatinine, Serum	0.7		mg/dL	0.5-1.5	OM
BUN/Creatinine Ratio	17			8-27	OM
Sodium, Serum	143		mmol/L	135-148	OM
Potassium, Serum	4.4		mmol/L	3.5-5.5	OM
Chloride, Serum	102		mmol/L	96-109	OM
Carbon Dioxide, Total		36 H	mmol/L	20-32	OM
Calcium, Serum	9.1		mg/dL	8.5-10.6	OM
Protein, Total, Serum	7.0		g/dL	6.0-8.5	OM
Albumin, Serum	3.9		g/dL	3.5-5.5	OM
Globulin, Total	3.1		g/dL	1.5-4.5	OM
A/G Ratio	1.3			1.1-2.5	OM
Bilirubin, Total	0.5		mg/dL	0.1-1.2	OM
Alkaline Phosphatase, Serum	66		IU/L	25-150	OM
AST (SGOT)	23		IU/L	0-40	OM
ALT (SGPT)	14		IU/L	0-40	OM
LIPID PANEL WITH LDL/HDL RATIO (FINAL)					
Cholesterol, Total	163		mg/dL	100-199	OM
Triglycerides	46		mg/dL	0-149	OM
HDL Cholesterol	59		mg/dL	40-59	OM
VLDL Cholesterol Cal	9		mg/dL	5-40	OM
LDL Cholesterol Calc	95		mg/dL	0-99	OM
LDL/HDL Ratio	1.6		ratio units	0.0-3.2	OM

```
              LDL/HDL
            Men  Women
1/2 Avg.Risk 1.0  1.5
   Avg.Risk 3.6  3.2
 2X Avg.Risk 6.3  5.0
 3X Avg.Risk 8.0  6.1
```

OM	Providence Med Grp DBA Mobile PHONE	CONTACT	DIRECTOR
	6701 Airport Blvd Ste A101 (251) 633-8880		G Divittori MD
	Mobile, AL 366080000		

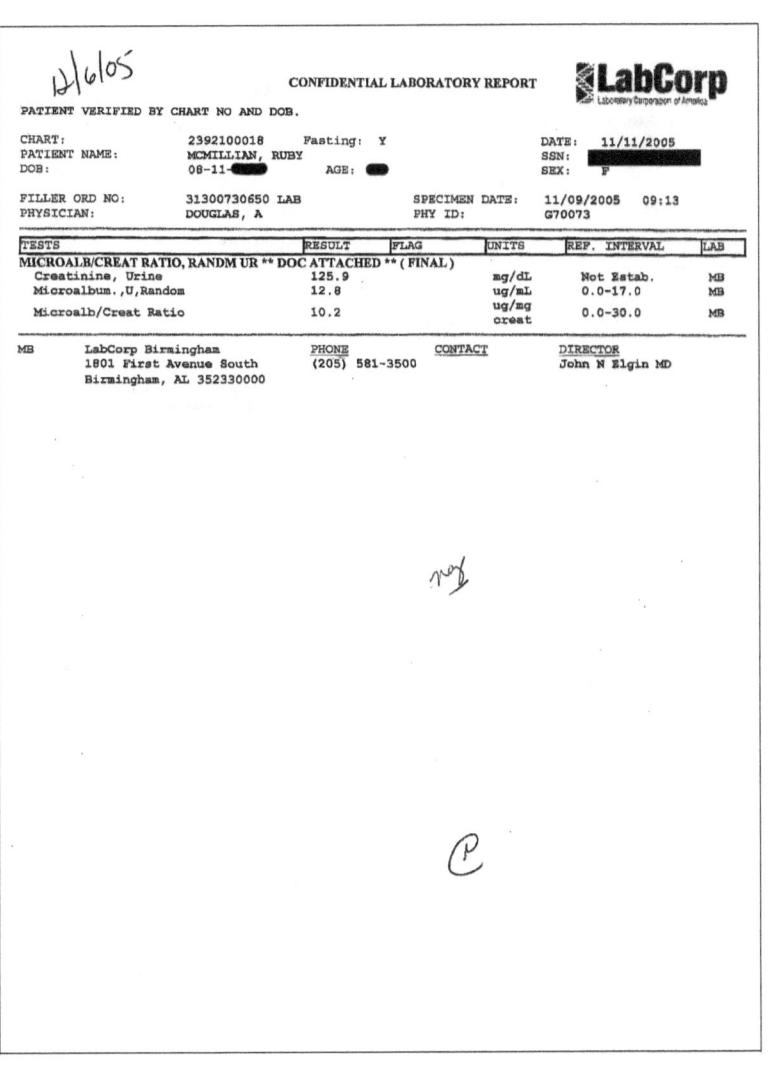

12/6/05

CONFIDENTIAL LABORATORY REPORT

LabCorp
Laboratory Corporation of America

PATIENT VERIFIED BY CHART NO AND DOB.

CHART:	2392100018	Fasting: Y		DATE:	11/11/2005
PATIENT NAME:	MCMILLIAN, RUBY			SSN:	
DOB:	08-11-	AGE:		SEX:	F

FILLER ORD NO:	31300730650 LAB		SPECIMEN DATE:	11/09/2005 09:13
PHYSICIAN:	DOUGLAS, A		PHY ID:	G70073

TESTS	RESULT	FLAG	UNITS	REF. INTERVAL	LAB
MICROALB/CREAT RATIO, RANDM UR ** DOC ATTACHED ** (FINAL)					
Creatinine, Urine	125.9		mg/dL	Not Estab.	MB
Microalbum.,U,Random	12.8		ug/mL	0.0-17.0	MB
Microalb/Creat Ratio	10.2		ug/mg creat	0.0-30.0	MB

MB	LabCorp Birmingham	PHONE	CONTACT	DIRECTOR
	1801 First Avenue South	(205) 581-3500		John N Elgin MD
	Birmingham, AL 352330000			

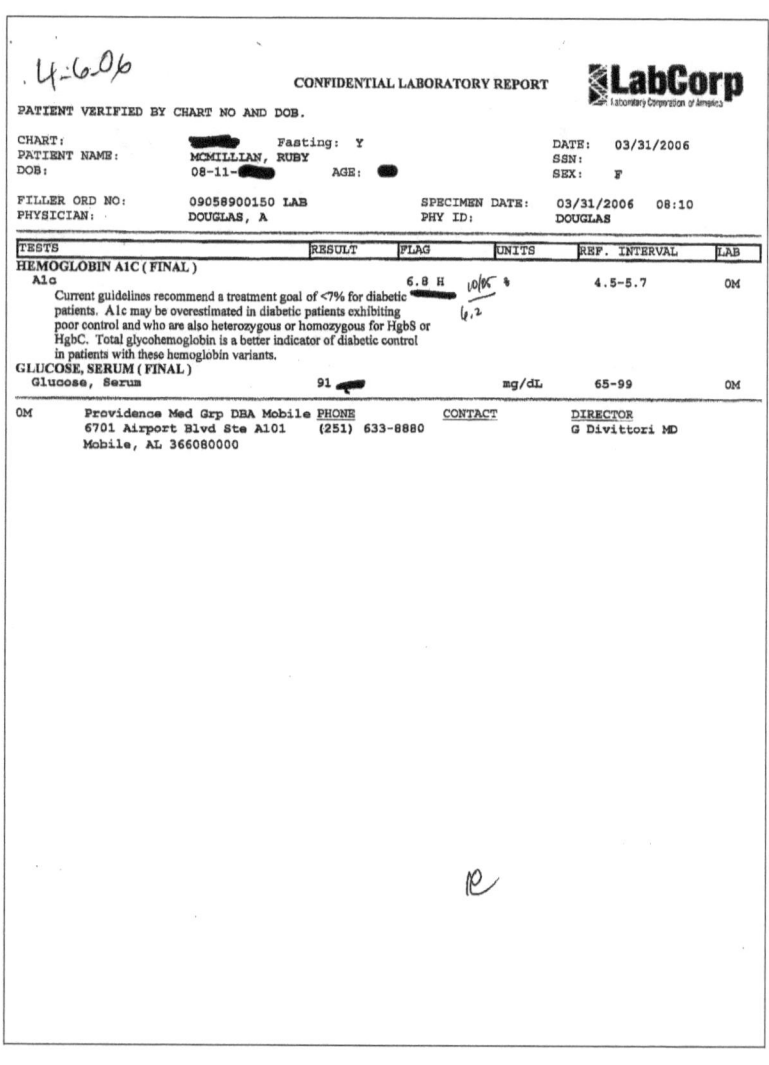

4-6-06

CONFIDENTIAL LABORATORY REPORT

LabCorp
Laboratory Corporation of America

PATIENT VERIFIED BY CHART NO AND DOB.

CHART:	Fasting: Y	DATE: 03/31/2006
PATIENT NAME:	MCMILLIAN, RUBY	SSN:
DOB:	08-11-█████ AGE: ███	SEX: F

FILLER ORD NO:	09058900150 LAB	SPECIMEN DATE:	03/31/2006 08:10
PHYSICIAN:	DOUGLAS, A	PHY ID:	DOUGLAS

TESTS	RESULT	FLAG	UNITS	REF. INTERVAL	LAB
HEMOGLOBIN A1C (FINAL)					
A1c	6.8 H	*10/05* %		4.5-5.7	OM

Current guidelines recommend a treatment goal of <7% for diabetic
patients. A1c may be overestimated in diabetic patients exhibiting
poor control and who are also heterozygous or homozygous for HgbS or
HgbC. Total glycohemoglobin is a better indicator of diabetic control
in patients with these hemoglobin variants.

GLUCOSE, SERUM (FINAL)					
Glucose, Serum	91		mg/dL	65-99	OM

OM	Providence Med Grp DBA Mobile PHONE	CONTACT	DIRECTOR	
	6701 Airport Blvd Ste A101 (251) 633-8880		G Divittori MD	
	Mobile, AL 366080000			

FOUR MAJOR AREAS OF OBSERVATION FOR TYPE - 2 DIABETES PREVENTION: ⮞

CONFIDENTIAL LABORATORY REPORT **LabCorp**
Laboratory Corporation of America

PATIENT VERIFIED BY CHART NO AND DOB.

CHART: 239210 Fasting: DATE: 03/29/2007
PATIENT NAME: MCMILLIAN, RUBY   SSN:
DOB: 08-11-█ AGE: █   SEX: F

FILLER ORD NO: 08858900440 LAB   SPECIMEN DATE: 03/29/2007 08:34
PHYSICIAN: ,   PHY ID: DOUGLAS

TESTS	RESULT	FLAG	UNITS	REF. INTERVAL	LAB
COMP. METABOLIC PANEL (14) (FINAL)					
Glucose, Serum	83		mg/dL	65-99	OM
BUN	9		mg/dL	5-26	OM
Creatinine, Serum	0.7		mg/dL	0.5-1.5	OM
BUN/Creatinine Ratio	13			8-27	OM
Sodium, Serum	137		mmol/L	135-148	OM
Potassium, Serum		5.7 H	mmol/L	3.5-5.5	OM
Chloride, Serum	100		mmol/L	96-109	OM
Carbon Dioxide, Total		33 H	mmol/L	20-32	OM
Calcium, Serum	9.6		mg/dL	8.5-10.6	OM
Protein, Total, Serum	6.9		g/dL	6.0-8.5	OM
Albumin, Serum	4.0		g/dL	3.5-5.5	OM
Globulin, Total	2.9		g/dL	1.5-4.5	OM
A/G Ratio	1.4			1.1-2.5	OM
Bilirubin, Total	0.4		mg/dL	0.1-1.2	OM
Alkaline Phosphatase, S	55		IU/L	25-150	OM
AST (SGOT)	20		IU/L	0-40	OM
ALT (SGPT)	12		IU/L	0-40	OM
LIPID PANEL WITH LDL/HDL RATIO (FINAL)					
Cholesterol, Total	140		mg/dL	100-199	OM
Triglycerides	34		mg/dL	0-149	OM
HDL Cholesterol	49		mg/dL	40-59	OM
VLDL Cholesterol Cal	7		mg/dL	5-40	OM
LDL Cholesterol Calc	84		mg/dL	0-99	OM
LDL/HDL Ratio	1.7		ratio units	0.0-3.2	OM

LDL/HDL
Men Women
1/2 Avg.Risk 1.0 1.5
Avg.Risk 3.6 3.2
2X Avg.Risk 6.3 5.0
3X Avg.Risk 8.0 6.1

HEMOGLOBIN A1C (FINAL)					
Hemoglobin A1c ▬	▬6.4 H (4.8)			4.8-5.9	OM

3/04

Current guidelines recommend a treatment goal of <7% for diabetic patients.

OM   Providence Med Grp DBA Mobile PHONE   CONTACT   DIRECTOR
6701 Airport Blvd Ste A101   (251) 633-8880   G Divittori MD
Mobile, AL 366080000

Susan~ total Cholesterol 6-5-10
Fax = 866-787-6860

CONFIDENTIAL LABORATORY REPORT

LabCorp
Laboratory Corporation of America

I# 39691

PATIENT VERIFIED BY CHART NO AND DOB.

CHART:	2392100018	Fasting: Y	DATE:	12/08/2008
PATIENT NAME:	MCMILLIAN, RUBY		SSN:	
DOB:	08-11-	AGE:	SEX:	F

FILLER ORD NO:	34358900360 LAB	SPECIMEN DATE:	12/08/2008 09:07
PHYSICIAN:	ANG, R	PHY ID:	

TESTS	RESULT	FLAG	UNITS	REF. INTERVAL	LAB
COMP. METABOLIC PANEL (14) (FINAL)					
Glucose, Serum	89		mg/dL	65-99	OM
BUN	13		mg/dL	5-26	OM
Creatinine, Serum	0.7		mg/dL	0.5-1.5	OM
Glom Filt Rate, Est	>59		mL/min/1.73	>59	OM
If African-American	>59		mL/min/1.73	>59	OM
Note: Persistent reduction for 3 months or more in an eGFR <60 mL/min/1.73 m2 defines CKD. Patients with eGFR values >/=60 mL/min/1.73 m2 may also have CKD if evidence of persistent proteinuria is present. Additional information may be found at www.kdoqi.org.					
BUN/Creatinine Ratio	19			8-27	OM
Sodium, Serum	139		mmol/L	135-145	OM
Potassium, Serum	4.2		mmol/L	3.5-5.5	OM
Chloride, Serum	103		mmol/L	97-108	OM
Carbon Dioxide, Total	31		mmol/L	20-32	OM
Calcium, Serum	8.7		mg/dL	8.5-10.6	OM
Protein, Total, Serum	6.7		g/dL	6.0-8.5	OM
Albumin, Serum	3.8		g/dL	3.5-5.5	OM
Globulin, Total	2.9		g/dL	1.5-4.5	OM
A/G Ratio	1.3			1.1-2.5	OM
Bilirubin, Total	0.5		mg/dL	0.1-1.2	OM
Alkaline Phosphatase, S	51		IU/L	25-150	OM
AST (SGOT)	17		IU/L	0-40	OM
ALT (SGPT)	9		IU/L	0-40	OM
LIPID PANEL WITH LDL/HDL RATIO (FINAL)					
Cholesterol, Total	145	145	mg/dL	100-199	OM
Triglycerides	59	28	mg/dL	0-149	OM
HDL Cholesterol	75	71	mg/dL	>39	OM
According to ATP-III Guidelines, HDL-C >59 mg/dL is considered a negative risk factor for CHD.					
VLDL Cholesterol Cal	12		mg/dL	5-40	OM
LDL Cholesterol Calc	58	71	mg/dL	0-99	OM
LDL/HDL Ratio	0.8		ratio units	0.0-3.2	OM
HEMOGLOBIN A1C (FINAL)					
Hemoglobin A1c	5.9	58	%	<7.0	OM
Diabetic Adult <7.0					
Healthy Adult 4.8 - 5.9					
(DCCT/NGSP)					
American Diabetes Association\'s Summary of Glycemic Recommendations for Adults with Diabetes: Hemoglobin A1c <7.0%. More stringent glycemic goals (A1c <6.0%) may further reduce complications at the cost of increased risk of hypoglycemia.					

OM   Providence Med Grp DBA Mobile PHONE   CONTACT   DIRECTOR

Copy to PT

CONFIDENTIAL LABORATORY REPORT   ▓LabCorp
Laboratory Corporation of America

PATIENT VERIFIED BY SSN AND DOB
PLEASE VERIFY CHART NO.

CHART:		Fasting:	DATE: 04/14/2010
PATIENT NAME:	MCMILLIAN, RUBY		SSN:
DOB:	08-11-██	AGE: ██	SEX: F

FILLER ORD NO:	10458900340 LAB	SPECIMEN DATE:	04/14/2010 08:22
PHYSICIAN:	DOUGLAS, A	PHY ID:	G70073

TESTS	RESULT	FLAG	UNITS	REF. INTERVAL	LAB
COMP. METABOLIC PANEL (14) (FINAL) 322000					
Glucose, Serum	86		mg/dL	65-99	OM
BUN	11		mg/dL	5-26	OM
Creatinine, Serum	0.81		mg/dL	0.57-1.00	OM
eGFR	>59		mL/min/1.73	>59	OM
eGFR AfricanAmerican	>59		mL/min/1.73	>59	OM

Note: Persistent reduction for 3 months or more in an eGFR
<60 mL/min/1.73 m2 defines CKD. Patients with eGFR values
>/=60 mL/min/1.73 m2 may also have CKD if evidence of persistent
proteinuria is present. Additional information may be found at
www.kdoqi.org.

BUN/Creatinine Ratio	14			8-27	OM
Sodium, Serum	140		mmol/L	135-145	OM
Potassium, Serum	4.4		mmol/L	3.5-5.5	OM
Chloride, Serum	103		mmol/L	97-108	OM
Carbon Dioxide, Total	28		mmol/L	20-32	OM
Calcium, Serum	8.9		mg/dL	8.7-10.2	OM
Protein, Total, Serum	6.9		g/dL	6.0-8.5	OM
Albumin, Serum	3.8		g/dL	3.5-5.5	OM
Globulin, Total	3.1		g/dL	1.5-4.5	OM
A/G Ratio	1.2			1.1-2.5	OM
Bilirubin, Total	0.4		mg/dL	0.1-1.2	OM
Alkaline Phosphatase, S	47		IU/L	25-150	OM
AST (SGOT)	20		IU/L	0-40	OM
ALT (SGPT)	7		IU/L	0-40	OM
LIPID PANEL WITH LDL/HDL RATIO (FINAL) 235010					
Cholesterol, Total	171		mg/dL	100-199	OM
Triglycerides	61		mg/dL	0-149	OM
HDL Cholesterol	81		mg/dL	>39	OM

According to ATP-III Guidelines, HDL-C >59 mg/dL is considered a
negative risk factor for CHD.

VLDL Cholesterol Cal	12		mg/dL	5-40	OM
LDL Cholesterol Calc	78		mg/dL	0-99	OM
LDL/HDL Ratio	1.0		ratio units	0.0-3.2	OM

CONFIDENTIAL LABORATORY REPORT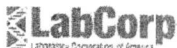

PATIENT VERIFIED BY CHART NO AND DOB.

CHART:	239210	Fasting: Y	DATE:	04/15/2010
PATIENT NAME:	MCMILLIAN, RUBY		SSN:	
DOB:	08-11-	AGE:	SEX:	F

FILLER ORD NO:	10400730490 LAB	SPECIMEN DATE:	04/14/2010	08:35
PHYSICIAN:	DOUGLAS, A	PHY ID:	G70073	

TESTS	RESULT	FLAG	UNITS	REF. INTERVAL	LAB
MICROALB/CREAT RATIO, RANDM UR ** SEE ATTACHED MR239210 ** (FINAL) 140285					
Creatinine, Urine	187.4		mg/dL	15.0-278.0	MB
Microalbumin, Urine	13.6		ug/mL	0.0-17.0	MB
Microalb/Creat Ratio	7.3		mg/g creat	0.0-30.0	MB
VITAMIN D, 25-HYDROXY (FINAL) 081950					
✳Vitamin D, 25-Hydroxy ✳	29.5 L		ng/mL	32.0-100.0	MB

Recent studies consider the lower limit of 32.0 ng/mL to be a
threshold for optimal health.
Hollis BW. J Nutr. 2005 Feb;135(2):317-22.

MB	LabCorp Birmingham 1801 First Avenue South Birmingham, AL 352331935	PHONE (205) 581-3500	CONTACT	DIRECTOR John Elgin MD

FOUR MAJOR AREAS OF OBSERVATION FOR TYPE-2 DIABETES PREVENTION: ⅄

HEMOGLOBIN A1C (FINAL) 001453

Hemoglobin A1c		5.7 H	%	4.8-5.6	OM
Increased risk for diabetes:	5.7 - 6.4				
Diabetes:	>6.4				
Glycemic control for adults with diabetes:	<7.0				

OM	Providence Med Grp DBA Mobile	PHONE	CONTACT	DIRECTOR
	6701 Airport Blvd Ste A101	(251) 633-8880		G Divittori MD
	Mobile, AL 366080000			

CONFIDENTIAL LABORATORY REPORT

☒ Laboratory Corporation of America

PATIENT VERIFIED BY CHART NO AND DOB.

CHART:	Fasting: N	DATE: 04/09/2011
PATIENT NAME:	MCMILLIAN, RUBY	SSN:
DOB:	08-11- AGE:	SEX: F

FILLER ORD NO:	09800730520 LAB	SPECIMEN DATE: 04/08/2011 07:50
PHYSICIAN:	DOUGLAS, A	PHY ID: 1528072113

TESTS	RESULT	FLAG	UNITS	REF. INTERVAL	LAB
MICROALB/CREAT RATIO, RANDM UR (FINAL) 140285					
Creatinine, Urine	163.5		mg/dL	15.0-278.0	MB
Microalbumin, Urine	6.7		ug/mL	0.0-17.0	MB
Microalb/Creat Ratio	4.1		mg/g creat	0.0-30.0	MB

MB	LabCorp Birmingham	PHONE	CONTACT	DIRECTOR
	1801 First Avenue South	(205) 581-3500		John Elgin MD
	Birmingham, AL 352331935			

FOUR MAJOR AREAS OF OBSERVATION FOR TYPE-2 DIABETES PREVENTION:

PATIENT VERIFIED BY SSN AND DOB
PLEASE VERIFY CHART NO.

CHART:	0023921000	Fasting:	DATE:	04/11/2011
PATIENT NAME:	MCMILLIAN, RUBY		SSN:	
DOB:	08-11-	AGE:	SEX:	F
FILLER ORD NO:	09858900390 LAB		SPECIMEN DATE:	04/08/2011 07:40
PHYSICIAN:	DOUGLAS, A		PHY ID:	1528072113

TESTS	RESULT	FLAG	UNITS	REF. INTERVAL	LAB
COMP. METABOLIC PANEL (14) (FINAL) 322000					
Glucose, Serum	84		mg/dL	65-99	OM
BUN	10		mg/dL	8-27	OM
Creatinine, Serum	0.71		mg/dL	0.57-1.00	OM
eGFR If NonAfricn Am	93		mL/min/1.73	>59	OM
eGFR If Africn Am	107		mL/min/1.73	>59	OM
Note: A persistent eGFR <60 mL/min/1.73 m2 (3 months or more) may indicate chronic kidney disease. An eGFR >59 mL/min/1.73 m2 with an elevated urine protein also may indicate chronic kidney disease. Calculated using CKD-EPI formula.					
BUN/Creatinine Ratio	14			11-26	OM
Sodium, Serum	140		mmol/L	135-145	OM
Potassium, Serum	4.9		mmol/L	3.5-5.5	OM
Chloride, Serum	103		mmol/L	97-108	OM
Carbon Dioxide, Total	31		mmol/L	20-32	OM
Calcium, Serum	8.9		mg/dL	8.6-10.2	OM
Protein, Total, Serum	6.8		g/dL	6.0-8.5	OM
Albumin, Serum	4.0		g/dL	3.6-4.8	OM
Globulin, Total	2.8		g/dL	1.5-4.5	OM
A/G Ratio	1.4			1.1-2.5	OM
Bilirubin, Total	0.4		mg/dL	0.1-1.2	OM
Alkaline Phosphatase, S	52		IU/L	25-165	OM
AST (SGOT)	17		IU/L	0-40	OM
ALT (SGPT)	7		IU/L	0-40	OM
LIPID PANEL WITH LDL/HDL RATIO (FINAL) 235010					
Cholesterol, Total	157	150	mg/dL	100-199	OM
Triglycerides	75	73	mg/dL	0-149	OM
HDL Cholesterol	77	71	mg/dL	>39	OM
According to ATP-III Guidelines, HDL-C >59 mg/dL is considered a negative risk factor for CHD.		stable			
VLDL Cholesterol Cal	15		mg/dL	5-40	OM
LDL Cholesterol Calc	65	64	mg/dL	0-99	OM
LDL/HDL Ratio	0.8		ratio units	0.0-3.2	OM
HEMOGLOBIN A1C (FINAL) 001453					
Hemoglobin A1c	5.8 H	5.7%		4.8-5.6	OM
Increased risk for diabetes:	5.7-6.4				
Diabetes:	>6.4				
Glycemic control for adults with diabetes:	<7.0				

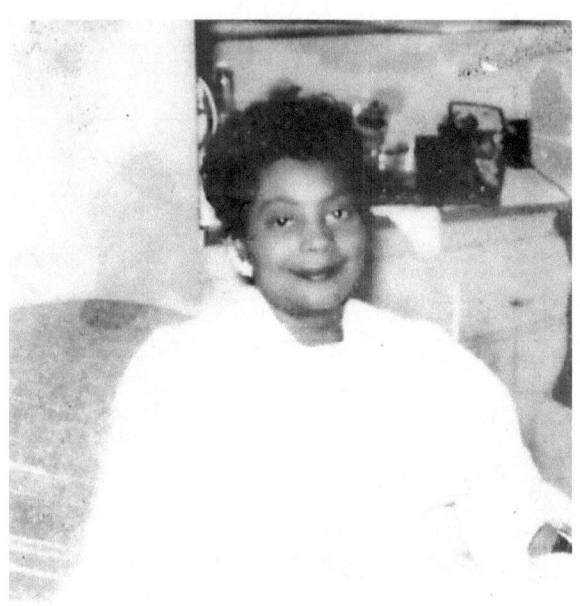

TO MY MOTHER: 1926- 1958

IT IS STILL HARD TO BELIEVE THAT YOUR PRESENCE STILL MAKES ME SMILE AFTER SOME 50 YEARS. THE FEW SHORT YEARS YOU SHARED YOUR LOVE WITH ME HAS NEVER LEFT.

AS AN ADULT, I UNDERSTAND BETTER HOW GOD'S LOVE IS FOR HIS CHILDREN. ALL THAT I HAVE GONE THROUGH WITHOUT YOU, SURELY HAS MADE ME THE WOMAN I AM TODAY. YOUR GRANDSON FONDLY CALLED YOU HIS ANGEL. IT WAS OK BECAUSE I KNEW YOU COULD HANDLE BOTH OF US.

MISS YOU, MOMMA

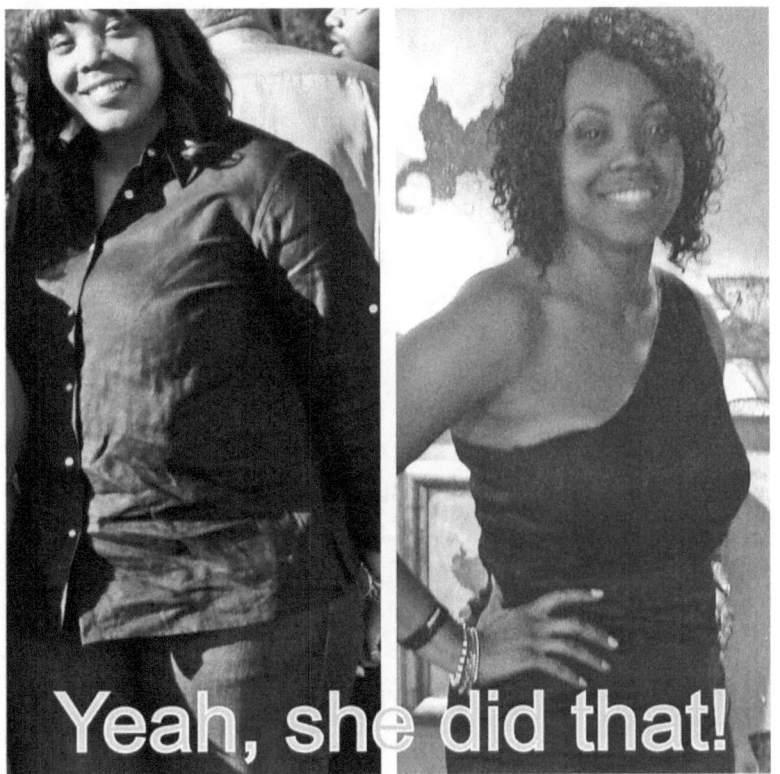

Yeah, she did that!

MY DAUGHTER-TOYIA

I NEEDED TO CHANGE MY LIFESTYLE AND EATING HABITS FOR LONGEVITY. BEING PREDISPOSED TO TYPE-2 DIABETES I KNEW I HAD TO MAKE A CHANGE. SOME YEARS AGO, MY MOTHER MODELED A HEALTHY LIFESTYLE CHANGE FOR ME. SHE OFTEN TALKED ABOUT THE "KINGDOM PRESCRIPTION". I DID NOT KNOW EXACTLY WHAT IT WAS BUT I SAW THE CHANGES IT MADE YEAR AFTER YEAR IN HER LIFE. THIS NEW LIFESTYLE HAD GIVEN HER A GREATER SENSE OF PEACE, CONFIDENCE, GRACE

AND STRENGTH. NOT TO MENTION A GREAT BODY AT 60-SOMETHING.

I HAVE WITNESSED THE DEVASTATION OF TYPE-2 DIABETES AND KIDNEY DISEASE IN THE LIVES OF MY LOVED ONES. MY DECISION WAS TO BE FIT FOR ME. MY DESIRE WAS TO DEVELOP A HEALTHY LIFESTYLE FOR MYSELF THAT I COULD LIVE WITH. THE KINGDOM PRESCRIPTION HAS PROVEN TO BE BENEFICIAL TO ME PHYSICALLY, EMOTIONALLY AND SPIRITUALLY.

NOW I CAN SHARE AND MODEL THESE HEALTHY HABITS WITH OTHER AFRICAN AMERICAN COMMUNITIES AS A MOTHER, DAUGHTER, SISTER, FRIEND AND MEMBER OF DELTA SIGMA THETA SOROITY INCORPORATED. THANKS, MOM, FOR BEING MY INSPIRATION.

I LOVE YOU, TOYIA

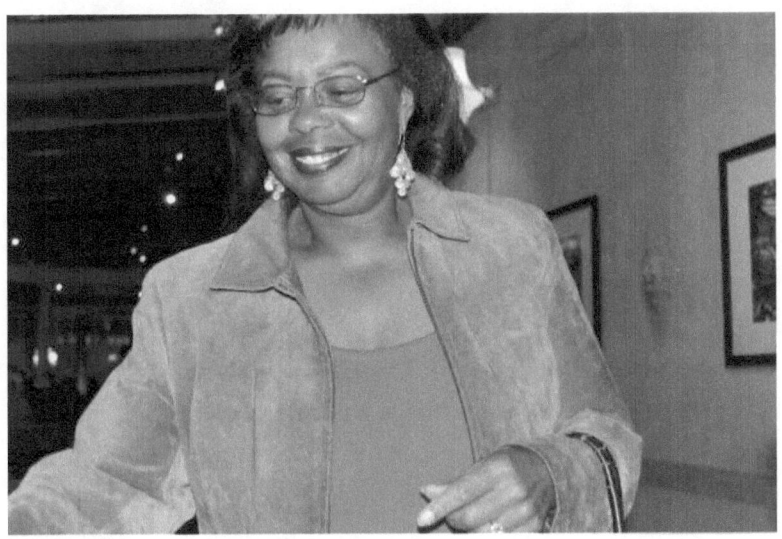

MY SISTER, MAGGIE-

YOU HAVE ALWAYS KNOWN THE RIGHT WORDS TO SAY TO MAKE ME FEEL SPECIAL. BUT TODAY I WANT TO THANK YOU FROM THE BOTTOM OF MY HEART FOR SAVING MY SON'S LIFE. DURING THE TIME THAT ROBBEN WAS IN THE HOSPITAL LYING HELPLESS IN A COMA, YOU PRAYED AND KEPT ME ENCOURAGED.

AFTER HE REGAINED CONSCIOUSNESS YOU BECAME HIS MINISTER AND LIFE COACH. THANK YOU FOR SHARING AND MODELING THE "KINGDOM PRESCRIPTION" LIFESTYLE WITH HIM. IT LITERALLY SAVED HIS LIFE. I WILL NEVER BE ABLE TO EXPRESS TO YOU MY GRATIUDE. I KNOW THAT YOU ARE GOING TO HELP THOUSANDS OF OTHERS TOO. YOU ARE MY HERO!

-MAGGIE

MY STORY TOO

Like many others I have known about diabetes for some time. But also like you I did not do the things necessary for my body to be healthy. Just exactly what is Type- 2 diabetes? In simple terms: Type 2 Diabetes is a metabolism disorder. Metabolism refers to the way our bodies use digested food for energy and growth. Most of what we eat is broken down into glucose. This is where I will direct you to the information via the American Diabetes Association (ADA) website. Please visit: www.ada.org to gain the correct understanding of why some people become diabetic and others do not.

There are three types of diabetics. I want to talk with you explicitly about Type 2 Diabetes and especially how to rid your body of this disease. Yes, you can be diabetes-free! Yes, you can take control of it with the "Kingdom Prescription." First, I want to give thanks to God for these revelations. As I have tried them one by one I've learned the benefits of each component. Today I am living proof that it will save your life from the devastation of losing vital organs that this dreaded disease is known to destroy in your temple over time.

Here are some startling statistics from the American Diabetes Association on the number of reported new cases of Type 2 Diabetes each year. This disease can be asymptomatic and you feel no symptoms until it has done major damage to your body. If you know that your family has a generational history of "sugar" as it is commonly called, please get yourself checked. At this moment, you probably already know that you have been experiencing those sick feelings after you have had a big meal the day before. Sometimes you feel lethargic and have to take a nap after you have your meals.

This book has a mandate to share the "Kingdom Prescription" with the world. God so loved the world that he gave his only begotten Son, whosoever believeth on Him shall not perish but shall have everlasting life. Therefore, the Kingdom Prescription has been sent to set those that are bound by this disease free.

Here is where we prepare for the transition that is coming to change our lives forever.

The day I left the doctor's office I was mad at myself, teed-off and scared all at the same time. After walking to my car, I got in and threw my head back and said, "Father God, you are my creator, you know what I need to regulate my blood sugars. You know what I need to do to make permanent changes so I can live and not die! Lord, I am sorry for not honoring my body (your temple). I confess that I have had no discipline regarding what I put into my mouth. Lord, forgive me. I will not leave this earth before my time just because I gave my body everything except the nutrients that will keep it functioning like a fine tuned machine. In the name of Jesus, I know you have said that healing is the children's bread.

Help me! Help me to stay focused so I can keep this disease from overtaking me. I believe that as the creator of my life, I give you full rein to remake this temple that it might be fit for the master's use. Thank you for your recipes and prescriptions to heal and restore this body. I receive it in the mighty, match-less name of Jesus the Christ, Amen!

While I was driving home I was quiet and was listening for the Holy Spirit. It was within a few minutes that the Holy Spirit brought to my remembrance my pregnancy with my daughter. You had hyperglycemia signs then. But only at birth did you realize that you were starting to swell-up more often. I had pregnancy-induced diabetes and was not told until the last week of my pregnancy. That's why my labor was four days long and the delivery was so dry and hard. That is why your daughter only weighted 5 lbs. 8 0zs.

Also remember when you were pregnant with your son? With him you did not have pregnancy-induced diabetes but you did have a thyroid goiter. Remember you had to eat often with your son? Even after you had eaten you still needed to lie down and take a nap?

Remember, with your daughter your weight went from 165 lbs. to 235 lbs. at birth? You cried out to me at that time and I answered you. You did what I instructed you to do and your body returned back to its normal weight over a one-year period. During your second pregnancy you were very active, ate a grapefruit every other day, roller skated, took long walks and ate lots of peanut butter sandwiches with honey. During that pregnancy you gained a total of 28 lbs. At conception your weight was about 160 lbs. At the birth of your son your weight was 188 lbs. Your baby weighed 8 lbs. 5 ozs. He was 21 inches long. Your fluid gain was about 8 lbs. The after birth was another 3 lbs. So immediately after birth you only had about 10 lbs. of your pregnancy weight left. After six weeks you were back into your regular clothing. Follow these steps that I will give you and your body will be healthier than you have ever been before. Quietly within myself I said, "Yes Lord, thank you for your faithfulness toward me."

Below I've described how I developed this little book with the answers that will bring healing to your body within weeks.

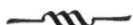

Being a healthcare provider for some 25 years, I knew about the problems diabetes caused. However, I have now experienced it up close and personal. I asked God to show me what to do for his temple to keep it free from this dreaded disease. I vowed that over the next three years, I would research scripture and natural solutions to rid my body of this silent killer. Here is the beginning of my prayerful journey as I read the Word of God about diseases.

Deuteronomy 28: 60-61 says this, "Moreover He will bring upon you all the diseases of Egypt, which thou was afraid, and they shall cling to you. Also every sickness and every affliction which is not written in this Book of this Law, the Lord will bring upon you until thou are destroyed." I then cried because it was very harsh. As I sat in silence for a while I began to understand that this was all due to disobedience. Disobedience is not just in disobeying His Word in our walk with him but also disobeying Him in how we treat our bodies which are his temple.

After my second outcry the Holy Spirit asked me this question.

Do you not know that your body is the temple of the Holy Spirit? I turned to 1 Cor. 6: 19-20 and it says this, "Do you not know that your body is the temple (the very sanctuary) of the Holy Spirit Who lives within you, Whom you have received (as a gift) from God? You are not your own. You were bought with a price (purchased with a preciousness and paid for, made His own). So then, honor God and bring glory to Him in your body."

In this experience, I knew that the Holy Ghost had arrested me. My body was in a state of disease because I did not have authority, discipline nor a consistent commitment to caring for what He has given me. I prayed, "Help me to stay focused and change my appetite to the things that are best for my temple."

Again, I looked at the Word for God's design for his temple. I went to the beginning in the Word in Genesis 2:7 says this, "And the Lord (Jehovah-The Existing One) God (elohim-The True God)) formed man of the dust of the ground, and breathed into his nostrils the breath of life; and man became a living soul. I also did a word study of this verse in the Hebrew. Here is the revelation of the text. Our God (formed) meaning a divine creation full of purpose. God made man an original individual design. God used the powered dust of a specific ground. It was red ground that was to be a yielding sustenance for our nourishment. Man was to look reddish in color. Then God blew boiling and soothing breaths into the nostrils.

Here is where God showed me that there are two types of breathing. One is to create and congeal the inner parts of man. The second one is the Breath of Life. This word "Breathe" in the Hebrew (05397) means (Nesh-aw-man) The Spirit of God. This Hebrew word primary means (Nasham) to pant as a woman in travail or labor. Life (02416) Chay/Khahee means "a living sustenance." Webster says that Sustenance is a sustainment; support; means of livelihood.

It is that which sustains life with food and nourishment. Therefore, we can only have this breath of life by spiritually inhaling his Word on a daily basis. Without his Word being our daily breaths, our bodies will be formed but our souls will be without the sustenance of the His Holy Spirit.

Let us look at soul in this text. Soul in the Hebrew means (nephesh) the inner being of a man or woman. The soul is where the seat of our will is; it is our character which is dubious. Our emotions can then sometimes make our character questionable, skeptical and even doubtful.

CHAPTER 5

Know Your "Type 2" Numbers

It has taken me almost thirty years to get the complete understanding of just how important it is for me to know the meaning of my blood work lab results. My metabolic panel lab report gives me a clear view of how my blood and electrolytes are doing. One specific aspect of this test is called my Hemoglobin A1C. This is the test that determines if I am in a pre-diabetic state or if I have become an insulin-dependent diabetic. Knowing your metabolic numbers here will save your life. The average healthy A1C is 4.8-5.6. Increased risk of diabetes the numbers are 5.7-6.4. In the pre-diabetes stage your numbers are 6.4- and above. Full blown/insulin-dependent diabetic is when your numbers are 7.0 and above.

Diabetes has taken a place in the lives of many African American families. According to the American Diabetes Association research, African American families are at a risk of some 13.3 % higher than other ethnic races to have this disease. These facts, along with my personal list, I have to tell our people how to live a healthier lifestyle. Why? Death is the premature enemy waiting for those who continue to be unaware of the importance of knowing their own metabolic numbers. These tests are taken every three months.

According to Jordan Rubin, author of "The Great Physician's Rx," he defines diabetes as a chronic degenerative disease caused by the body's inability to either produce enough insulin or properly use insulin, which is essential for the proper metabolism of blood sugar, also known as glucose." Here is how I personally define diabetes, DI-A-BETES as the proclaimed silent killer of the temple of God (your body). The word alone denotes that something is to die. Di-a-betes causes your body to slowly start killing your vital organs without giving you warning. Ask your doctor to explain to you how diabetes works on your vital organs. Long before you experience any symptom of diabetes, it is at work in your body. Here is an easy and precise way you can start tracking your numbers.

During your annual visit to the doctor you have blood work done. Ask for a copy of your lab results to take home. LOOK at your numbers on the lab report. You will see several columns. They are listed as the following: TEST, RESULTS, FLAG UNITS REF. INTERVALS AND LAB. (I have given you a copy of my lab report) I do know that all lab reports are not categorized the same. In the Ref. Interval column there are numbers that are commonly called, within normal limits. For example, Glucose serum norms are 65-99. I always try to keep my numbers between 80-90. Another vital area to look for is your HEMOGLOBIN AIC. This gives you an accurate account of how your blood sugars average over the past three to four months.

Take a look at the numbers again for what is called normal.

Those numbers are 4.8-5.6. Increased RISK for diabetes are 5.7 -6.4. You have DIABETES when your numbers are 6.4. The last category is the glycemic control for adults with diabetes is 7.0. So if your numbers (metabolic panel) are not within normal limits you are in great danger of shortening your life. I am writing this book prayerfully with the body of Christ in mind. We must stop and honor the great gift of our bodies. It is the only temple we will have this side of heaven.

It is vital that we know how important our health is. We can have all the money we need and more but without good health we will see others reap the benefits of our hard work or inheritance. Look at 3 John 2 which says, "Dear friend, I pray that you may enjoy good health and that all may go well with you, even as your soul is getting along well. (NIV DSB). Here is where we have to stop, understand, take action and make small changes to realize optimum health. By going for a thirty-minute walk five days per week will literally help you shed pounds of unhealthy weight. Try eating at fast food establishments only one time per week instead of every other day.

I do know that first it takes a willing mind to make life changes. But when we know that we have a family history of diabetes, high blood pressure, obesity, blindness and heart attacks; it is our signal to make sure that we do not become the next victim. If we know that a thing will harm us or kill us and we take no actions for our own protection we will surely succumb to death. Poor health will cause us to not have the good life spoken of in 3 John 2.

Here is where the Word of God brought clarity and consistency to my irregular healthcare habits. Look at 1 Corinthians chapter 6 verses 19 and 20, which asks a specific question. "Do you not know that your body is a temple of the Holy Spirit, who is in you, whom you have received from God? You are not your own; V.20 you were bought at a price. Therefore honor God with your body…"

Our body is unique in that God made us in His image. We are fearfully and wonderfully made. You must realize and understand that you are the temple of the Holy Spirit that represents the church here on earth. You are the house of God that holds the greatest gifts with the ability to share it right here on earth with others. That is why we should reverence our bodies. It is important what we put in this vessel. Let us look at the scenario of owning a Rolls Royce. Just the name immediately denotes integrity, distinction and class. You would not take this car to Jiffy Lube to have it serviced. This vehicle requires a trained, certified technician to just change the oil. In other words, it takes a specialist to care for it because it has customized features inside and out.

Is not your human body more valuable than a Rolls Royce? Yes, it is! Because we are, why do you keep taking it to places that give you cheap oil in exchange for your money? Like a valuable automobile it requires a "special auto care program." It means that we have to purpose to make some life changes. We can make better choices of our food. Food is our fuel or our debris. Look at some of the best fuel foods available.

One Day of Great Fuel Foods
Breakfast:

    ½ cup Old-fashioned oatmeal
    ½ cup Great Grains, crunchy pecans cereal
    1 tsp. cinnamon,
    1tsp. of vanilla flavor
    12 raisins
    1/4 cup of chopped walnuts,or (¼ cup of granola)
    1/4 tsp. of Sea salt

Put this in a bowl and stir together. Pour in one cup of water to 2/3. Place in the microwave for two minutes. Stir after two minutes. Put in a pat of real butter and stir. Return to microwave for the last 30 seconds.

Now add 1/4 cup of low-fat milk or non-fat milk and stir and eat! If you want a real treat add two tablespoons of International coffee creamer-French Vanilla. This is high octane for your body. Having this high fiber breakfast just three times per week would help your elimination problems. Note: Breakfast is one of the most important meals of your day. Drink a bottle of water.

Mid-morning snack: 1-gala apple or a fruit-flavored yogurt. Drink a bottle of water.

Lunch:

Try a quarter of baked juicy chicken (white or dark) and a salad.

If you prefer to have a "liquid lunch" try a low sodium soup with wheat crackers and a cup of fruit. If you have time on the days that you have a liquid lunch go for a brief 15-minute walk. Drink a bottle of water. You can also do some stretching and chair exercises at your desk if 75% of your day is spent in front of a computer. Just remember that it is the small consistent movements that will get long term results.

Dinner: by 6:00 p.m.

Why? The later you eat and do not walk at least fifteen minutes briskly you will wear it to bed. Unused calories late in the evening will turn into fat. Try a great stir-fry of fresh vegetables: washed and chopped onions, squash, broccoli, celery, cauliflower, greens and a medium-sized baked sweet potato. Add fish, chicken or lamb if you need a meat alongside your stir-fry. Drink a bottle of water.

As you read further, I am going to share my personal health regime. But it is absolutely vital that you understand the importance of the fact that what you put inside your temple will be the direct result of how it will perform for you. Rethink your future with a health mindset. Say this out loud right now, "My body is my most valuable machine." This is one of my objectives for writing this book; it is to encourage you to keep your temple free of the disease (dis-ease) called diabetes. I am speaking specifically about keeping healthy kidneys, avoiding CVA'S, a stroke caused by continued extreme high blood pressure, avoiding those extreme highs and lows emotionally and avoiding those sudden feelings of being sick to your stomach accompanied by sweats, rapid heartbeat and nervous shaking. Avoid those awful leg cramps and feeling hungry again a couple of hours after you have had a meal.

I was tired of not having enough energy to concentrate on anything for a long period of time. The one that I'm still working through is having a nasty, snappy attitude or demeanor with everybody when my sugar is spiraling down. This means that I need to eat or drink something right now before I pass out. Those of you who have experienced these moments of hypoglycemia (low blood sugar) know what I mean. Sometimes these are often followed by severe headaches and the need for a quick nap. Of course as soon as you eat or drink something you have an urge to go to the bathroom. Is this the kind of life you want to live on a regular basis? Think on this, if your automobile would do these things to you on your way to work in the morning wouldn't you get it to the repair shop ASAP?

Having the right tools to fix the problem is the key. Here are a few tools to help you get started and keep your body operating at its optimum performance levels. It is in the bloodstream. Chromium, calcium and magnesium are three trace minerals that simply help the body work in harmony. Why are these three so important? Chromium acts like insulin in the body. Magnesium helps promote a healthy pancreas and helps stop those bad leg cramps. Calcium helps build great bones, hair and teeth.

After the doctor told me that I was a diabetic in 2007 and gave me a prescription for diabetes I made up in my mind at that moment that the disease called diabetes will not kill me. This killer called diabetes today would be arrested by the Holy Spirit that indwells me. I acknowledged that this was my own doing. I had allowed my temple to be defiled because I conformed to this world's standard of eating and not exercising on a regular basis. I asked the Holy Spirit to forgive me for not offering my body as a living sacrifice, holy and acceptable unto the Lord which I know is my reasonable responsibility of worship. When I did this, I started crying in my car outside in the parking lot.

As I sat there, I went over and over in my mind the lessons that I had learned in medical assisting training. I thought about the two doctors that taught me while in ex-termship training at Visitation Valley Family Practice in San Francisco, California in 1981. They recognized that I was very hyper-active and sometimes quick to give answers that were sharp without the intention of being rude. The doctor approached me with a lab report on some of his patients. He explained to me that blood work will always determine what your body currently has working in it; while it will also tell you what it needs to correct the problem.

As we went through a few of these lab tests I focused on the column that showed me what was within normal limits. I asked if they would do blood work on me for free. He laughed and asked me what I was looking for? I answered nothing special just wanted to have a look at my own lab results. When the lab work was completed the doctor brought my results to me. He said, "During lunch let's look this thing over OK?"

At lunch the doctor pointed out a few high level numbers concerning my cholesterol, my A1C, my lack of calcium and magnesium. That was the time I began working with the doctor to rid my body of all the clogs that had brought me to this point. My God has made me fearfully and wonderfully. It was then that I asked God to help me start honoring my temple in the way it was meant to operate.

I was determined to decree and declare that the spirit of sugar di-a-be-tes would stop its curse on my family. This curse had taken members of my family long enough. It had claimed two of my great-aunts, my father, my eldest brother and sister: the latest was my son, Taurius.

This does not have to be your story. Look at what I call the super mix for a balanced health performance. Doing the kingdom prescription will help you to achieve and maintain a healthy and balanced lifestyle. It is in the doing that makes the difference.

CHAPTER 6

30 Days Preparation for Success:

Make a list of the things you need to pick up at the store to get you started right.

1. Always check with your doctor before making changes due to medication.

2. Get supplements/vitamins.

3. Purchase your food. Get as many super foods as possible.

4. Get your blood sugar meter/strips/diary

5. Design your week to have three to four days of physical exercise for 30-40 minutes.

6. Weigh yourself the first thing in the morning. Tell the truth! Take your measurements: hips, waist and chest area.

7. Ask someone to hold you accountable for these new changes for four weeks.

8. Weigh yourself after the 30 days. Take your measurements. Take your blood sugar and tell us your numbers now.

9. Practice the "Breath of Life Treatments." Start with the count of five holding after you exhale instead of eight counts.

10. Every 21 days your body renews the blood. Your first 30 days will mark your next month's success. Give yourself the gift of NEW BLOOD!

SPIRITUAL TOOLS: READ AND DECLARE THE WORD

1. SCRIPTURE: 3 JOHN 2 (NIV) Dear friends, I pray above all that you may enjoy good health and that all may go well with you, even as your soul is getting along well.

2. SCRIPTURE: 1COR. 6: 19-20, (NIV) Do you not know that your body is a temple of the Holy Spirit, who is in you, whom you have received from God? You are not your own; V.20 you were bought with a price. Therefore honor God with your body.

Websites for more information:

www.BiblicalHealthInstitute .com

www.crosswalk.com

CHAPTER 7

Type 2 Diabetes Questionnaire-Test Yourself

Name, _____

1. Explain in your own words how diabetes makes you feel:

   _____

   _____

2. How many times per day do you drink water?

   _____

3. What are some of your favorite foods?

   _____

   _____

4. Is there a history of diabetes in your family?

———————————————————————————

What is your blood pressure?

———————————————————————————

5. Do you check your blood sugars?

———————————————————————————

What are your normal levels?

———————————————————————————

6. What are some of your favorite types of exercises/ movements?

———————————————————————————

———————————————————————————

7. What is your AlC number?

———————————————————————————

8. Do you have any current sores or breaks on your body?

———————————————————————————

Where?

———————————————————————————

Describe it:

_____

_____

9. How much do you currently weigh?

_____

How much do you want to weigh in 90 days?

_____

10. Do you have regular check-ups?

_____

11. Do you take any vitamins/minerals currently?

_____

12. Are you willing to go through the transformation to rid your body of Type 2 Diabetes?

_____

Date: _____

Score: _____

CHAPTER 8

"Great Food Ideas"

In the scheme of making our lives over into the new and divine, we must make our food consumption be the best ever. This is our sure place to restructure. This is the place of grace in our search for what will ultimately satisfy our taste buds and put a smile on our face. Food is an art, a fuel, a family affair and the thing that brings people together more than anything else. Here is where you need to give yourself permission to change. Break out of the traditions that have caused our bodies to become ill. Declare that you will accept the "new thing" God is giving you in your appetite.

During the next 30 days thank God for His personal prescription that will cause you to make a permanent change.

Change is when you make a conscious choice to do things differently regardless of what it takes. Renew the spirit of your mind with this revelation about the word change.

The Holy Spirit impressed upon my heart what God wants from us in this change. (Acronym). Hear this today in the Spirit.

C-Clearly

H-Hearing

A

N-Need

G-God

E-Expresses

Now that we understand that our bodies are His vessel to do the work for Him on earth, God's desire has been expressed. Can you now make a permanent change with his help?

Here we are ready to locate, cook, taste and combine some of the best combinations of food that the earth has to offer us. I believe that the best types of food for our bodies are those foods that provide a healing component--foods that are valuable in digestible enzyme nutrients. We need foods that give our bodies a healthy dose of fiber to guarantee our proper elimination on a daily basis.

Stop and take inventory of what God provided for us to eat from the Garden of Eden before all the additives and pesticides. Think of food as a rainbow of colors. They have a specific reason for their colors. Green vegetables are full of chromium and antioxidants. Remember you just learned that our bodies need chromium a trace mineral that helps your body mimic insulin production. Foods like broccoli, spinach, cabbage, brussels sprouts, romaine lettuce, avocados, granny apples, leeks, all the herbs, onion, red and green bell peppers.

The yellow /orange groups are full of vitamin C. Some of the foods are yellow summer squash, yams, yellow peppers, carrots, acorn squash, onions and melons. Purple group are rich in beta-carotene.

Look at blueberries, eggplant, purple onions and peppers and various fruits. Look at the many types of nuts and seeds. Nuts are rich in fiber and protein. When we eat a ½ cup to 1 cup of nuts it is o.k. to eliminate meat from that meal. We have a great array to choose from such as almonds, cashews, pecans, walnuts (Black), acorns, peanuts, pumpkin seeds, sunflower seeds, pistachio, macadamia and Brazil nuts. Make a beautiful rainbow of your own personal delight with some of your favorites.

SMOOTHIES

Here is one of my favorites whole food drinks that I make when I want to go liquid for one meal or for a 24 hour period. When I use this method as my only food intake during a 24 hour period it allows me to get quite, read the Word of God and pray without missing the nutrients my body needs. During my liguid fast I also drink lots of Green Tea sweetened with a little Agave Nector.

Smoothies can be a quick and easy way to give your body a blast of green, yellow, orange and blue super foods in one glass. My person machine of choice is the Magic Bullet.

Smoothie Blast

8 oz. glass
¼ cup of crushed ice
2 oz. of Aloe Vera juice
2 oz of Apple juice
¼ cup blueberries
8 to 10 Almonds/unsalted
1 scoop of Green Protein Powder
½ small banana

Put on the cap tight, shake and put on the bullet. 30 to 45 seconds. Enjoy!

Veggie Smoothie

8 oz glass
¼ cup crushed ice
2 oz of Aloe Vera juice
1 hand full of washed spinach
¼ of a small washed fresh beets
2 slices of pineapple packed in its own juice
3 small baby carrots

Put the cap on tight, shake and put on the bullet for 45 seconds. If too thick you can always add some water to reach the consistency you desire.

OILS TO "LIVE" BY

OLIVE OIL: An old ancient oil that has healing and cleansing properties for our bodies. Olive Oil is rich in mono-unsaturated fats. Use it for cooking your favorite dishes. Use about four tablespoons in a non-stick pan to prepare your Stir-fry or blackened Meats. If you do not have Olive Oil use Peanut Oil, Flax Seed Oil or Sesame Seed Oil. Here's a recipe for one of my all time favorites.

Mrs. Ruby's Chicken-N-Veggie.

Try this stir-fry for 6 to 8 servings.

4 boneless chicken breasts or boneless chicken thighs.
1 large purple onion
2 large green/yellow/orange bell peppers
4 large carrots
1 large raw broccoli floret Or 1 large bag of frozen broccoli
16 oz. can of Campbell (Low-Sodium) Cream of chicken or Broccoli & Cheese or Cream of Mushroom
2 tablespoons of Olive Oil

Preparation:
Wash chicken and pat dry

Cut into strips- one half to one inch—set aside in a bowl with cover on it. (BOWL OF COOL WATER FOR THE VEGGIES)

Veggies: carrots-wash with veggie brush/cut off top and bottom. Cut into thin angled slices.

Bell Peppers: wash, cut off top, take out seeds and membrane. Cut into good bite size chunks.

Onion: Cut off top and bottom, peel. Cut into nice size chunks.

Raw Broccoli: rinse off. Cut stem into bite size pieces. Cut the top Floret in half. Cut again into good bite size pieces.

Cooking Instructions:

Heat a large non-stick pan on top of stove/medium heat. Make sure pan is hot—add 2 tablespoons of Olive Oil

Add chicken-lightly pepper (Use black or white)

Use a wooden spoon to stir the chicken around for about 8 to 10 minutes. (Make sure the chicken is completely done).

Empty cooked chicken into a deep roasting pan. Set aside.

There is usually some juice from the chicken. Add 1 table-spoon of Olive Oil--heat. Add veggies- stir until soft but crispy (7 to 10 minutes) Put them in pan with cooked chicken.

Last item: Take ¼ stick of butter place in pan and stir-fry the big onion by itself/glaze only. (Just heat the onion until it all has touched the fire for 2 minutes or so). Put in pan with chicken and veggies

Add ½ can of Low Sodium-Campbell Cream of Chicken/or Broccoli Cheese or Cream of Mushroom.

Open the can of soup- stir ½ of the entire can into your pan of chicken and veggies completely. Mix well- Let stand for 10-15 minutes with a cover-Serve over Brown rice. (Great to make in advance-put in frig. Use as desired)

DESSERT:

Mix fresh fruit
Sponge cake or Angel Food Cake
Low-Fat Cool Whip

Top with Granola or sliced almonds (few)

Presentation: Place a nice slice of sponge cake on a dessert dish. Put a couple of spoons of fresh fruit on the cake, garnish with Cool Whip and sprinkle on granola or sliced almonds.

Drink: Fresh Lemonade

Juice of one lemon
1 quart of water
Use Agave Nectar to taste
Add the zest of fresh lime/ ½ of the peel

"Enough is Enough"

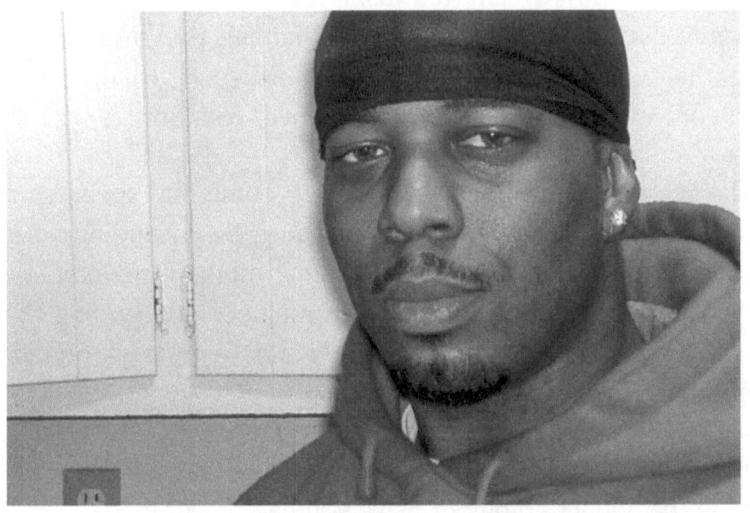

Dedicated to my Son, Taurius Jamahl Franklin
August 21st 1973 - March 23rd 2012

My day started out as usual. It was late in the month of February 2012. I walked my half-conscious body to the kitchen to get the first cup of coffee. Then I went to my favorite place in my home, my office/prayer room. As I took a few sips of coffee my mind began to work and focus on the things I needed to pray about. Our new business was about to start a new six-week class. I believed that this was the place and the time, for everything God had said was about to bust wide-open.

After about an hour of soaking in worship music and telling my God about everything I could think of, my soul felt better. I reached over to pick up my cell phone to check for messages that might have been left from the night before. Sure enough I had two from my son, Taurius. It read, "Hey, pretty lady, just wanted you to know that I am so thankful for you being my mother and being there for me all these years. Thank you for the prayers that have covered me. Love, your Son!

The second text read, "I want you to come and spend some time with me. Pack your bags because I am sending you a round trip ticket to Maryland." At that moment my emotions went a little to the south. My last memory of spending time with this boy in a place where I did not have my own room did not make me happy.

About 9:00 a.m. the phone rang and it was Taurius. "Hey Momma, what's going on? Have you had prayer yet?"

"Yes, I have."

"Can we pray before you go to the office?"

"Sure, how are you?"

"Trying to stay alive! Trying to get things up and running again. Did you get my text? I am so ready for you to come and see my house, Momma. It is so nice and the owner gave me a break to move in. Can we Skype later tonight?"

"OK, son, you know that I am getting ready for work. So let's pray when I get in the car. I will call you back in about ten to fifteen minutes OK?"

As usual I am a little slow in the mornings. But today, I had to make that 10:00 a.m. on time. Got my bag, purse and keys and off to the car. While waiting for the car to warm-up I called Taurius.

As he answered the phone his first words were, "Pray for my strength and the spirit of suicide to be lifted off me, Momma."

"Listen, Jamahl, let me say this loud and clear so you and the demonic whisper that is listening will have no more mis-understanding. Mr. Taurius Jamahl Franklin and the spirit of negative influence with demonic imps, everything that does not bring my baby boy a good report is a lie. You are cast down into the abyss where you belong. No weapon formed against my son shall ever prosper.

"Satanic attack, you are bound, chained and without a voice in Jesus' name! Let the joy of the Lord be your strength now and forever. My love for you today will give you a big hug un-til we see each other—stay blessed, giving and grateful. Got to go now; have the day we proclaimed and I will talk with you tonight about eight p.m. Love yah!"

After a long day at the office I was drained and ready for some quiet, not drama. You see my son was home most of the time now because his life had changed since 2006. After a near death experience with acute renal failure due to untreated hypoglycemia and hypertension, he was found by his friends who saved his life by getting him medical help. When he woke up in the hospital and learned what had happened he knew that his lifestyle was changed. No more cross country traveler, but now his weekly routine consisted of three treatments per week connected to a dialysis machine for three to four hours until he received a kidney transplant. This was very hard for someone who had never been sick or hospitalized before.

For several years, however, Taurius knew that we had a family history of diabetes, high blood pressure and heart attacks. We would talk about family history often because he wanted to know about his grandmother, Lillie Mae. Lillie Mae was my mother who died in 1958 suddenly from cardiac arrest due to a blood clot after having a hysterectomy. Some of Taurius' conversations would be about how he knew my mother was his angel. But being a young man he felt that his body was in-destructible and he did not have to worry because he worked out and took protein shakes and vitamins. But he did learn that history will repeat itself if you do not take proper care of yourself.

It was about 8:15 when the phone rang. "Hey, are you ready to see my new place?"

"Yeah, give me a minute to hook up."

"How was your day, Ma?"

"Mine was good. I cooked me some stir-fried veggies with skinless chicken breast, sweet potatoes and some Snapple. It was off the chain. Wish you could have been here to see me prepare it--you would have been proud. Got your computer up?"

"Here we are, Momma. Take a virtual tour of my new place. Doesn't it look a lot like your office? I chose black and glass with some black and grey furniture. What do you think?"

"Jamahl, you did good, real good!"

"I am ready now to settle down and stay awhile in this house. Mom, you have to come and visit me. The owner is young and very nice. I told him about you and how long you've been in real estate."

"Son, you don't understand that I can't just drop everything and come to Maryland and spend a week. I have obligations here in Mobile."

"You are your own boss, right? I am going to pay for your flight and everything, Mom. I want you to just come and spend some quality time with me."

"OK, I want you to think about coming to Mobile and spending Easter with us. It is just you. Look into getting your doctor to arrange for you to have dialysis for two weeks here.

Your house is beautiful. Take some pictures and send them to me. You have arrived. I hope this is your home for a long time, Jamahl. Stay put and stop moving every year or so."

"Yeah, Mom, this is it for me."

"All righty then, it is time for me to go to bed. We can talk more tomorrow. Love yah."

Over the next week my old cell phone started to break-up really bad. I was talking to Taurius on the phone and it cut out again. When we did connect again he said, "It is time for another phone, Momma."

"Yes, you're right, so when are you going to send me one? I will not hold my breath because I know that you lie about money so I will get one over the next week or so. (We both laughed). Today, I am going to Western Union and wire you $225.00 to buy a phone.

"Sure Jamahl! You are my only point of consistent contact."

"They will call you when it arrives."

"OK, thanks Jamahl."

One time he did exactly what he said. Later that day I did receive the money and purchased a phone. For the next few weeks we were able to talk without any problem. Of course, my daily routine became first again. I noticed that every day he would put entries on his Facebook page. It was always giving thanks for another day and declaring that the love of God is real. One of the most memorable said, "God is soooooo good! He keeps doing it for me every day."

In mid-March, I felt a release of the past in the voice of Jamahl. He said, "Momma, I love you so much. I mean it!"

I said, "I love you too."

"Mom, I do not want to come to Mobile this month. I want to come for Easter so I will not be alone for the holidays."

"OK, get it cleared with your doctor."

"Oh, by the way, Mom, there is a new bus called Mega-Bus that can bring me there for twenty dollars. Yes, they have a special and I am going to ride in comfort."

It was about March 21, 2012 when we had a hit or miss phone call. So I texted him and said, "Let's pray in the morning. Love, Mom."

About 8:00 a.m. or so Taurius called me and said, "Momma, I need you to pray for me especially this week. I have a few things I need to do but I need strength. I am going to dialysis but I need to hear you pray.

I said, "I need to hear you sing to me. Practice what you preach." We both laughed. "Alright, let's go to the throne room."

Our Prayer & Song

Father God, in the name of Jesus we come to give you thanks, praise and glory for the things you have done for us to experience the liberty whereby Christ has set us free. We acknowledge that you are our Jehovah-Rohi, the God that heals. We acknowledge that you are Jehovah-Shalom our peace. We acknowledge that you are El-lohim our Father, Son and Holy Spirit.

Go with my son today and allow him to be wrapped in your protection and divine presence as he takes dialysis. I know that your word tells us in Mark 11: 24 these promises: therefore whatever we desire when we pray, believe that we have received it and it shall be. Right now we both agree with your word. Let the peace of God surpass all of Jamahl's understanding in Jesus name, Amen!

On the night of March 22nd about 9:00 p.m. I got a text just as I was turning off my cell for the night. It was Jamahl texting me, "Can you talk with me now?"

My whole being was tired and I felt like I could talk with him in the morning when I felt refreshed. Early the next morning I decided that I would call him and talk awhile before we prayed together. I texted him first and I waited for 15 to 20 minutes with no response. Then I called him and the phone went to voicemail.

I am thinking, "Well, since I didn't speak to him last night when he wanted me, this morning he is not answering." I went on with my quiet time. As I was praying, suddenly I started to hear the song by Walter Hawkins, "I'm Going Away" and "What is This?" At first I simply listened and smiled and hummed along with it. Later that day, I had planned to share the quiet time experience with Jamahl. This was a Wednesday morning. About 2:00 p.m. or so that afternoon I called his cell again. Left him a message that said, "Look Jamah, this is your Momma. you had better pick up that phone and call me and stop the silent mode. I was too tired to talk with you last night. Call Me, I love you."

By Friday morning I had had enough of the silence. So I sent him a text. "Son, why have you stopped communicating? Don't allow anything to keep you from calling me. Pick up the phone and call me or text me. Love yah, Mom."

I left and went to the office to finish out the week. But in the middle of lunch I heard the song again, "What Is this that makes me feel so good inside? What is this that just keeps setting my soul on fire, whatever it is, it won't let me hold, hold my peace..." That's why I'm going away, away oh! Yes, I am. I'm going to see Jesus, I gonna see my Savior's face. It won't be long. I'm going away-a--way oh! Yes, I am."Within myself I smiled. I had one more counseling session to complete at 1:00 p.m. During the latter part of this session my cell vibrated twice. During counseling I make it a habit of not taking calls. On the third vibrate I was moved to look at the numbers. I put the phone down and thought, I do not recognize these numbers.

I told the client I felt a need to pray so can we close our session because someone has called three times?As soon as I finished praying, the phone rang again. This time I answered. The voice on the other end asked, "Is this Reverend Ruby McMillian? I said, "Yes, it is. Who is calling?"

The next questions shook me when he asked if I was Taurius Franklin's mother. My first thought was, "Lord, what has this boy done now?"

I said, "Yes, who's calling?"

He said, "Mama, this is the Maryland Police department. Reverend McMillian, are you possibly driving or alone?"

I said, "No, I am not driving but I'm in my office alone. However, I am not alone in the building.

"Sir, could you tell me what my son has done please? Or, better yet, could you put him on the phone?"

He said, "Mama, I wish I could tell you some other way."

"Tell me what? Could you just put my son on the phone? Let him tell me. I have been trying to reach him for the past three days."

Then he asked, "Are you sitting down?"

Then I knew that something was very wrong. I asked him if he was with my son and he said yes.

"Reverend McMillian, I am so sorry but we have just found Taurius here at home and the paramedics could not do anything to help him at this time."

I asked, "What are you saying? Is he alright?"

The voice said, "Mama, I am so sorry but Taurius has passed away, apparently in his sleep. His phone was open to your picture by his side; that is how we were able to locate you so quickly. The Baltimore Humane Society will contact you."

"Oh, God! Oh, God! What are you saying? No! No! No, put him on the phone. God No! Not now! Not yet! Lord Jesus. God help me."

The voice in the phone said, "Mama let me get your address. Please tell me where you are so I can send you some help."

During my yelling, the receptionist came into my office. What's wrong? Are you sick? What's going on, pastor?"

"Take the phone, take the phone." During the process she got all the information and gave him our location.

All I can remember is that I felt like my breath was still. My voice was quiet. I called my husband. I vaguely remember calling my daughter. I said, "Baby girl, I have to talk to you for a few minutes."

She kept saying, "Momma, speak up. I can barely hear you. Momma, speak louder." Finally I said, "They found Jamahl. They found Jamahl, and they couldn't help him. He's gone, He's gone! Jesus help us."

She said, "What? Where is he? Momma, do you mean he's dead." Her voice went off. "Get somebody, Get somebody" is all I could think to say.

As I was being taken from the floor of my office, I looked up and an old college friend of mine from Covington Theological Seminary was holding my hand. He looked in my face and said, "I am here with you. I am here with you."

Soon my husband walked into my office and I lost it all. They put me in the truck and John brought me home and put me on the sofa. I called my pastor to come and pray with me. The next thing I remember is that we were praying and the pain was so great until I bent over forward. I thanked him and he went on his way.

It was about 4:00 a.m. in the morning when there was such a presence near me. I felt so near that I thought, Father God, thank you for the angel of mercy that will comfort me this night.

Just then the songs started again with much more clarity. This time it was different in the sequence in which it was heard. It was "I'm going away Oh! Yes I am. Whatever it is I just want to sing and shout—this time there is no one here to put me out. I want to see Jesus, I want to see Jesus. Thank you, Lord. I am going away (very slow)-I am going away."

As I sat and listened to these songs I broke through and asked the Holy Spirit to reveal to me the meaning. If there was something that was wrong with my sons' death, please show me. After prayer, I felt at peace. About 6:00 a.m. on Saturday morning I started searching for air fares to Maryland. About 8:00 a.m. I started trying to find the police officer that found my baby boy. I wanted to know all the details. It was Saturday and it was difficult to locate anyone because of the weekend.

On Friday, while I was out of my mind dealing with the news of my son, Amanda, the receptionist, wrote down the information on a card for me. On Saturday morning when I re-read the card again I realized that there was another name of a person to contact. He was the owner of the house. During the process somehow my daughter located the name and phone number of the owner. We did speak and what a pleasant voice. I was assured that everything would be kept until I arrived.

Mr. Greg made arrangements to pick me up at the airport on Monday at 5:00 p.m. What a joy it was to meet the person who was so pleasant on the phone. After getting the luggage in the car and getting settled in I couldn't wait to start asking questions. At that moment he suggested that I try to reach the officer that actually found Taurius. I got on the phone to try again and, to my surprise, I did reach him.

The officer did explain what he found when he arrived. But the thing that touched me the most was when he told me that this was his first experience with this type of discovery. "Mrs. McMillian, all I could do was pray. When I saw the phone I knew he was trying to make a final communication with you. I am so sorry for your loss. I felt better when the Chaplain arrived and was able to assist you."

"Sir, would you please just describe to me what you found? As he went through the details my heart was beating out of my chest. Oh God! Help me to stay together. After about five minutes of silence on the phone, a gentle hand touched mine and I looked into the eyes of Mr. Greg. My heart flooded over with tears and all I could say was "Jesus!" I thanked the officer for taking the time to explain everything to me. The officer said, "Mrs. McMillian, can we pray before we hang up?"

I said, "Please, would you?"

As the officer was praying my heart released more hurt. At the end of the prayer we both said amen. "Mrs. McMillian, if you need anything else please give me a call."

I said, "Thank you again, officer," and we hung up.

Mr. Greg asked, "Are you hungry? Let me say that I do not have any food at that house. What do you have a taste for? Please let me buy you something."

He took me to a Mexican place that was one of his favorite spots. This was a good time for us to get to know each other. I learned that he had a daughter named "Musu."

"Tell me, what does that name mean?"

He said with that big smile on his face said, "Little woman."

I shared that I also have a daughter named Toyia. "My daughter has given me three grandchildren. You will get an opportunity to meet part of my family tomorrow night." After dinner we were off to the house. My heart went to my throat again as I walked into the house.

Mr. Greg said, "Here is Taurius' room and the key .You can go in when you get ready. I put all the things in my room and went into Taurius' room. I sat in his office chair, looked around at all of his things. The color scheme of the room was black, grey and cream walls as his background. There was a beautiful bed, night stand, dresser and TV entertainment center where a

42-inch plasma TV sat. The walls were covered with pictures of the family.

I turned around in his office chair and looked at his meticulously arranged office space. The desk was glass, L-Shaped, with two tiers and grey steel frame. On top of the desk was a black surround sound system, a desk light, laptop in the center with a printer on the side of the desk. There was a black/grey art-deco rug on the floor.

As I took a deep breath, I started hearing the songs again. This time, what is this that makes me feel so good inside? Whatever it is it just won't let me hold my peace. It makes me love my enemies and it makes me love my friends and it won't let me be ashamed to tell the world that I've been born again!

My eyes, heart and soul were full of tears at the reality that my baby boy was not here. He is not going to come back to say to me, "Hey pretty lady."Later that evening about 10:00 p.m., I went to my room to try to get some rest. But about 2:00 a.m. the songs started again. It was so overwhelming that I sat up in bed and said, "Lord! This is too much for me. Please reveal to me if there was a wrongful thing in my sons' death? If it is something you want to reveal keep on singing. But if my Son is alright –give me your peace that will surpass all of my understanding in Jesus' name. I lay down again, drifted off to sleep and slept like a baby.

The next morning about 9:00 a.m. I made my way down to the kitchen for coffee. It was there that I met two of the roommates that shared the house with Taurius. Everyone gave me their sincere sympathy for my loss. They too were devastated at the loss of Taurius. As I sipped on my mug of coffee one of the guys said, "Taurius was planning for the two of you to have a great visit here. He talked about how much you had taught him about being organized so he wanted to show you that he heard you." I got up from the table and looked outside for a few moments trying to stop the tears.

There sat his new toy which he had named, "BIG BOI." It was his 2001-BMW-740IL. What a day we had over the phone as he made the purchase. I went back to my chair and told them the story. The truth be told I was very upset that the boy bought the car. I said, "Taurius, this is a used car salesman's dream come true. To see a young man with cash to blast out in a long 2001 BMW!"

He said, "Mom, you told me to always get the car-fax, have it checked out by an auto mechanic and negotiate a low ridiculous price, right?"

"Yeah! That's right."

"OK! I did that, so can I buy what I have always wanted, Momma? It has only had one owner, 110K miles and no wrecks or major body damage."

At that point I said, "OK, Jamahl! Call and get a quote from your auto insurance company and ask about the cost of a short-term auto warranty and add it to the cost of the cash price. He said, "Momma, I have already done that! But I want you to speak with the owner of the company. I could hear him speaking to the owner as he gave him the phone.

He said, "Sir, this is my financial advisor. Please give her all the stats about the car. If she says yes, it is a go! If she says no-I will walk away."

At that moment I simply laughed out loud! Mr. Greg came in and asked, "Mrs. Ruby, are you OK? Oh! Yeah, just reflecting on the car outside and how my baby boy lived in this beautiful place in New Carrolton, Maryland."

As he sat and joined us at the table; we had lots of laughs and woes about some of the stories that were shared about Taurius. Suddenly, it was some two hours since we took a break from reflecting on the days Taurius walked through the house as a self-appointed property manager for Mr. Greg. It was a good session for everyone because we left the table with a few less hurts and a few big hugs.

Mr. Greg and I stayed and talked about picking up the other family members from the airport. Mr. Greg did his best to instruct me how to get to the airport. He gave me a sheet that had directions from the front door of the house to the entrance of the airport. However, I am thinking, You do not know that I can get lost in the middle of the day. I know that I will make it but when is another matter. Due to Mr. Gregs' work schedule it was not possible for him to accompany me to the airport.

After a shower and another nap I was ready to revisit Taurius' room again. This time I was able to examine the surroundings for personal papers. In about an hour or so I left his room and went downstairs to watch TV until it was time to make the drive to the airport. It took me about one hour and 45 minutes to make it there. It was good to see my daughter Toyia, my sister, Maggie, and my nephew, Robben.

Thank God for technology on a little i-phone. My daughter asked me for the address to the house? With the help of the navigator on the i-phone we were able to make the return trip in 45 minutes. Everyone got inside to get settled after the long trip. We had a chance to talk about what we had to do to get Jamahl.

The very next morning we started the process of getting Jamahl from the state Humane Society. After speaking to the officials at the Humane Society I knew that I had a few lessons to learn. In the midst of the pain, I was in a new place and dealing with the state laws concerning an individual that was found deceased without any relatives in town or nearby. The coroner's office was not sure of the actual cause of death so state law required that the body must be frozen until the body was claimed by the family. My very gut went sore because I knew then that I would never see my baby boy again or hear him call me "pretty lady."My daughter, Toyia, worked untiringly to complete the obituary for Taurius' homegoing. The words were simply beautiful. After they were completed the entire family was off to New York for the day. Let me say this, I was not at all in agreement with this suggestion initially. But as I look back on it, I am truly glad that Toyia pressed to do something with the family so we could have memories that were not only focused on the death of Jamahl. Thank you, baby girl, from the bottom of my heart for making the "Homegoing Celebration" for Jamahl more enjoyable.

On April 9th 2012 at 6:00 p.m. we all gathered at Taurius'

favorite place in the house—the living room. It was a beautiful and intimate service. Our opening song was I Believe. I
offered a prayer and we all repeated the 23rd Psalm. At my
request, Toyia sang "Amazing Grace." Afterwards, everyone
had a few remarks about the joys and sometimes the misun-
derstood Taurius. There were plenty of laughs and moments
of silence. As I eulogized my baby boy, using Psalm 23. As
I shared my scripture, I talked about the days we spent together and how happy Taurius was. His days were filled with
sending e-mails, texts and posting on Facebook about the
goodness of God. Because we know that Taurius knew Jesus
for himself.

We will all trust that God knows the day and the hour that He
would bring Taurius home to live with him forever. I shared
with the family about the songs that were ringing in my heart
and soul. Two of Taurius' favorite songs were by Bishop Walter
Hawkins entitled, 'I'm going away' and 'What is this.' I believe
that Taurius is now singing these songs and dancing freely! He
is free from the burden and pain of weekly dialysis. He is free
from his regime of pills and restricted meals. I just want to
remind you that now Taurius is free to dance. Free to sing and
shout and there will be no one there to put him out!

He has gone away for now but one day we will sing and
dance together. He is free and free indeed in Jesus name! As I
closed this homegoing celebration about his life with us as we
know it; the Spirit of God prompted me to extend salvation to
all that were in the service.

Later in the week, my nephew said, "Thanks, auntie, for doing
such a great job for my boy. It has made me more thankful for

my own life. I was thinking about when I was in the hospital, almost dead, due to my diabetes being out of control.

Did I tell you, auntie, that the doctor told me that I had Type-2 Diabetes? Can you believe that just a few weeks ago I was in the hospital in a coma for three days? I could have died, man. auntie, I had to learn how to take care of myself and stop eating junk food all the time. I can't lie, it was hard at first.

But I started doing what you told me to do a long time ago. The more I walked, ate the baked fish, ate the baked chicken, ate the salads and watched my blood sugars, I needed less and less medicine. Right now, I only take two pills per day. No more needles for me. I have lost 45 lbs. auntie! But more importantly, thank you for helping me to reconnect with God. I love you auntie. That was worth the homegoing celebration for me to see and hear about a change that was taking place in my family to stop diabetes."

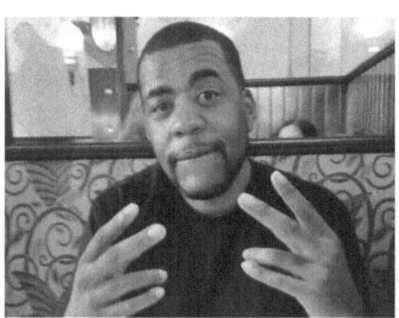

Now we were all focused on getting Toyia and Robben back to the Bay area. That day I was grateful for Maggie being with me. No one else could have filled that space. We got Toyia and Robben to the airport. On our way back it was time to prepare for our road trip to Alabama. Maggie stayed with me to make sure that "Big BOI" brought us safely home.

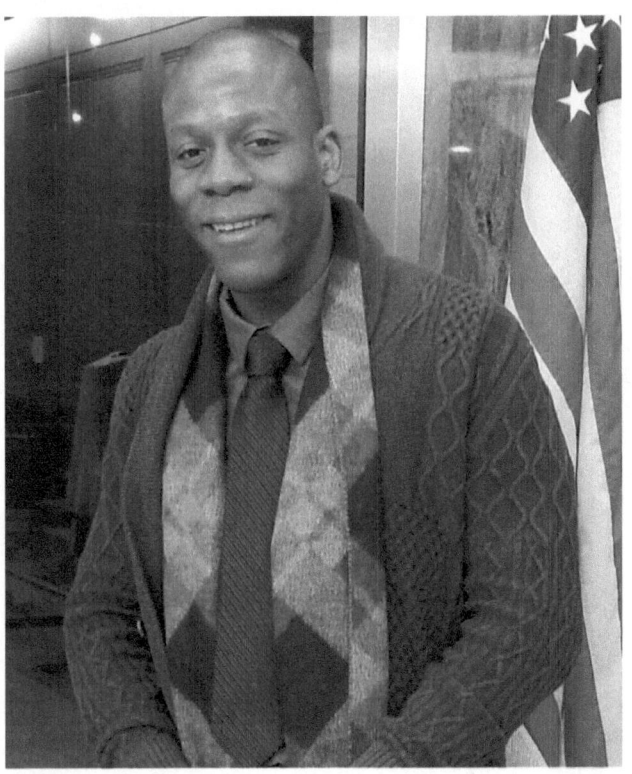

We all were forever grateful to the awesome hospitality that Mr. Greg extended to all of us. As a way of showing our gratitude we decided to redecorate a couple of the rooms in his home. Our hope is that it would remind him of us. This is my story that tells you why "Enough Is Enough". At the age of 37, my son Taurius slipped away from us simply because of unhealthy food and life choices. Learning the importance of good healthy food choices coupled with regular exercise will help anyone obtain long life. That is rich wisdom speaking!

This is why enough is enough for me. I have declared war on Type-2 Diabetes and kidney disease. Some 28 million people today have this disease. By the year 2030 that number could increase by a global two million. This disease can be reversed. Take an up close and personal look at your health. Have yourself tested at least twice per year, exercise daily and eat healthy. After all, you really only have one opportunity to live your best life now.

I knew the distinguished and acconpolished Mr. Taurius for a short period of time but, in that time I was and will forever be honored for the priviledge of knowing a man at the front linesof the fight against type2 diabetes with a cross in one hand, a bible in the other and the unwavering support and encouragement of his great family.

Mr. Taurius was more than just type2 diabetes. That was not his identity. He was a man with a genuine good heart, a desire and passion for knowledge that spoke with such conviction and ardor that you could feel his words.

From the first time we met our spirits connected and through conversation I could tell that he was altruistic and whatever he was involved in he rigorously approached it. Our interaction was through real estate and I developed confidence and penchant feelings towards him. This was a man that was and will foreverbe revered and extolled by many and due to his passing left many nostalgic. Just like in his life how he enchanced everyone he encountered he will do so in his passing vicariously through this book. Type 2 diabetes will end with me enough is enough!

The Common Touch
Empowerment Center

Purpose

Global Alert: There are literally thousands of new cases of Type 2 Diabetes being reported in the African community daily. Another sector in our community that is totally asymptomatic (do not feel sick) are our younger children. Thirdly, we are experiencing an epidemic of new juvenile diabetes cases that are increasing twice as fast as they did ten years ago. We need to wake-up and save ourselves by "Eating To Live."

OBJECTIVES: Bring these alarming numbers to the attention of the community. By using local television channels, interfacing with ADA Project Power, setting up classes of "How To Eat Yourself Healthy," to offer free testing for glucose, offer my personal book entitled "Diabetes Will Stop With Me". Hold weekly meetings with other community leaders so all people can learn how to be free of this "Silent Killer."

Personally, I know that by staying aware of your body blood work numbers you will have a healthier lifestyle and assist with setting the "Quick Start Program.

Future Local site: 3220 Rochester Dr. Mobile, AL. 36618, Renovation Cost: $100,000.00 (One-Hundred Thousand) to turn this site into a permanent headquarters to implement the following programs.

This will be a 2500 sq. ft. Community Center updated with four offices, commercial kitchen, community room, Exercise room and areas for meditation rooms. Our staff will be health professionals and volunteers that will take the hands-on approach to teach each individual how to become actively involved with their health. We will offer empower-ment tools to our community. Lives will be changed because the touch of Christ always gives us "New Life." This is an in-tegrated method that includes these components on a daily basis: prayer, eating super foods, physical movements and taking supplements that will assist your body to become well.

Benefits: Empower thousands yearly with the knowledge to understand about the "Silent Killer" named diabetes. Do what I was made to do: share with the world. Share the "Kingdom Prescription" that will reverse Type 2 Diabetes. If you want to be a part of the Empowerment Team-please visit our web site.

CONTACT: Rev. Ruby McMillian for speaking engagements, workshops and conferences.

Mailing address: P.O.Box 9002-Mobile, AL. 36691

Visit us on the web at www.thecommontouchinc.org.

E-Mail: thecommontouch@gmail.com.

Facebook: Ruby McMillian.

The Common Touch Empowerment Center

"THE KINGDOM PRESCRIPTION
THAT WILL REVERSE TYPE 2 DIABETES"

COURSE SYLLABUS

Instructor: Rev. Ruby McMillian

WEEK 1: YOUR BODY THE TEMPLE

1 Cor. 6; 19-20

Genesis 1:27 Your Image, Respecting yourself

Divine Health with integrated methods of wellness

WEEK 2: THE BREATH OF LIFE

Genesis 2:7

Isotonic Breathing Techniques Oxygenated Blood Benefits rid DIS-EASE Consistency of fifteen daily breaths

WEEK 3: THE BLOOD

Your Lab Reports

Know your numbers for your health's sake 90 day Glucose-Alc Blood Protein Extreme Makeover Journal your results

WEEK 4: SUPPLEMENTS/ FOOD PREPARATION

Natural supplements to lower blood sugars; Eating green, yellow, purple, red blue and lean. Design your success

Gifts of Movement- 1Cor. 12:4-9

Overview/ Questions

WEEK 5: PERSONALIZED PRESCRIPTION

Appointment-Schedule 30-minute consultation

All proceeds from the workshops will go to the renovation of 3220 Rochester Dr. Mobile, Al. This is the future Mobile Corporate Headquarters for "The Empowerment Center" due to open in the fall of 2013. Thank you for taking the steps to exchange the curse of the disease Type 2 Diabetes for life. Common Touch is a Charitable, Tax Exempt 501 (c) (3) Corporation.

Sponsored by the Kingdom Learning Institute

Healing Prayer

Father God, today is the first day for your children to take hold of this Kingdom Prescription Lifestyle in honoring their bodies as your temple. I ask that you grant them more grace where they are weak and wisdom where they lack it.

Today meet them at the point of their need. Just as I asked for your help in my time of sickness, you heard my cry and little by little you gave me strength and your peace.

I want to thank you, Lord, for what you have in store for your children during this stage of their transition. Holy Spirit, rule, reign and abide in each soul so they may know and experience you personally.

For these things we commit our bodies to you as a living sacrifice, holy and acceptable unto you, Lord, which we know to be our reasonable service. I receive this newness of life in Christ in Jesus' name. Amen

Healing Scriptures

Day 1

(Hosea 6:1, NKJV) "Come, and let us return to the LORD; For he has torn, but he will heal us; He has stricken, but He will bind us up."

Healing Scriptures

Day 2

(Jeremiah 33:6, NKJV) "Behold, I will bring it health and heal-ing; I will heal them and reveal to them the abundance of peace and truth."

Healing Scriptures

Day 3

(Malachi 4:2, NKJV) "But to you who fear my name The Son of Righteousness shall arise with healing in his wings; and you shall go out and grow fat like stall-fed calves."

Healing Scriptures

DAY 4

(Luke 18: 1 AMP) "Also Jesus told them a parable to the effect that they ought always to pray and not to turn coward (faint, lose heart , and give up)."

Healing Scriptures

Day 5

(Luke 6:19,18, AMP) "And all the multitudes were seeking to touch Him, for healing power was all the while going forth out of Him and curing them all (saving them from severe illness or calamities)."

(V.18) "Even those who were disturbed and troubled with unclean spirits, and they were being healed (also)."

Healing Scriptures

Day 6

(Luke 8:48, NKJV) "And He said unto her, 'Daughter, be of good cheer; your faith has made you well. Go in Peace'."

Healing Scriptures

Day 7

(Revelation 22:2, AMP) "Through the middle of the broad-way of the city; also, on either side of the river was the tree of life with its twelve varieties of fruit, yielding each month its fresh crop; and the leaves of the tree were for the healing and the restoration of the nations."

Healing Scriptures

Day 8

(Exodus 15:26, NKJV) "And saying "If you diligently heed the voice of the LORD your God and do what is right in His sight, give ear to His commandments and keep all His statues, I will put none of these diseases on you which I have brought on the Egyptians. For I am the LORD who heals you."

Healing Scriptures

Day 9

(Jeremiah 17:14, AMP) "Heal me O Lord, and I shall be healed; save me, and I shall be saved, for You are my praise."

Healing Scriptures

DAY 10

(Psalms 6:2, AMP) "Have mercy on me and be gracious unto me, O Lord for I am weak (faint and withered away); O Lord, heal me, for my bones are troubled."

Healing Scriptures

DAY 11

(Psalms 107:20, NKJV) "He sent his Word and healed them, and delivered them from their destructions."

Healing Scriptures

Day 12

(Matthew 4: 23, AMP) "And He went about all Galilee, teaching in their synagogues and preaching the good news (Gospel) of the Kingdom, and healing every disease and every weakness and infirmity among the people."

Healing Scriptures

DAY 13

(Luke 8:47, AMP) "And the woman saw that she had not escaped notice, she came up trembling, and, falling down before Him, she declared in the presence of all the people for what reason she had touched Him and how she had been instantly cured."

Healing Scriptures

DAY 14

(1 Corinthians 12:9, AMP) "To another (wonder-working) faith by the same (Holy) Spirit, to another, the extraordinary powers of healing by the one Spirit."

Healing Scriptures

Day 15

(Matthew 8:16, AMP) "When evening came, they brought to Him many who were under the power of demons, and he drove out the spirits with a word and restored to health all who were sick."

Healing Scriptures

Day 16

(Luke 17:15, NKJV) "And one of them, when he saw that he was healed, returned, and with a loud voice glorified God."

Healing Scriptures

Day 17

(Matthew 14:14, NKJV) "And when Jesus went out He saw a great multitude, and He was moved with compassion for them, and healed their sick."

Healing Scriptures

Day 18

(Isaiah 58:8, AMP) "Then shall your light break forth like the morning, and your healing (your restoration and the power of a new life) shall spring forth speedily; your righteousness (your rightness, your justice, and your relationship with God) shall go before you (conducting you to peace and prosperity) and the glory of the Lord shall be your rear guard."

Healing Scriptures

DAY 19

(Proverbs 4:20-22, AMP) "My son, attend to my words; consent and submit to my sayings. V21. Let them not depart from your sight; keep them in the center of your heart. V22. For they are life to those who find them, healing and health to all flesh."

Healing Scriptures

Day 20

(Psalms 147:3, AMP) "He heals the brokenhearted and binds up their wounds (curing their pains and their sorrows)."

Healing Scriptures

DAY 21

(Psalms 30:2, NKJV) "O LORD my God, I cried out to you, and You healed me."

Healing Scriptures

Day 22

(Matthew 10:8, AMP) "Cure the sick, raise the dead, cleanse the lepers, drive out demons. Freely (without pay) you have received freely (without charge) give."

Healing Scriptures

Day 23

(James 5:16, AMP) "Confess to one another therefore your faults (your slips, your false steps, your offenses, your sins) and pray (also) for one another, that you may be healed. Is any among you sick? He should call for the church elders (the spiritual guides). And they should pray over him, anointing him with oil in the Lord's name."

Healing Scriptures

Day 24

(Luke 5:17, NKJV) "Now it happened on a certain day, as He was teaching, that there were Pharisees and teachers of the law sitting by, who had come out of every town of Galilee, Judea and Jerusalem. And the power of the Lord was present to heal them."

Healing Scriptures

Day 25

(Matthew 8:13, NKJV) "Then Jesus said to the Centurion, 'Go your way; and as you have believed, so let it be done for you.' And his servant was healed the same hour."

Healing Scriptures

Day 26

(2 Chronicles 7:14, AMP) "If my people, who are called by My name, shall humble themselves; pray, seek, crave and require of necessity My face and turn from their wicked ways, then will I hear from heaven, forgive their sin, and heal their land."

Healing Scriptures

DAY 27

(Jeremiah 33: 2-3, AMP) "Thus said the Lord who made (the earth), the Lord who formed it to establish it –the Lord is His name: V 33. Call to me and I will answer you and show you great and mighty things, fenced in and hidden, which you do not know (do not distinguish and recognize, have knowledge of and understand)."

Healing Scriptures

DAY 28

(Proverbs 3:7-8, AMP) "Be not wise in your own eyes; reverently fear and worship the Lord and turn (entirely) away from evil.V8. It shall be health to your nerves and sinews, and marrow and moistening to your bones."

Healing Scriptures

DAY 29

(Mark 5:34, AMP) "And He said to her, 'Daughter, your faith (your trust and confidence in Me, springing from faith in God has restored you to health. Go in (into) peace and be continually healed and freed from your (distressing bodily) disease.'"

Healing Scriptures

Day 30

(1 Corinthians 6:19, AMP) "Do you not know that your body is the temple (the very sanctuary) of the Holy Spirit Who lives within you, Whom you have received (as a gift) from God? You are not your own."